W9-CWY-518

RETURNING TO SCHOOL

A Guide for Nurses

Donea L. Shane, R.N., M.S.
Assistant Professor
University of New Mexico
College of Nursing

PRENTICE-HALL, INC., Englewood Cliffs, New Jersey 07632

Library of Congress Cataloging in Publication Data
Main entry under title:

Returning to school.

Includes bibliographies and index.
 1. Nursing—Study and teaching—Psychological aspects. 2. Nurses—Psychology. 3. Nurses—Attitudes.
I. Shane, Donea L., (date). [DNLM: 1. Education,
Nursing, Continuing. 2. Nurses—Psychology.
3. Education, Nursing, Graduate. WY 18.5 S528r]
RT73.R45 1983   610.73'07   82-18124
ISBN 0-13-779165-8
ISBN 0-13-779157-7 (pbk.)

Editorial/production supervision and interior design by Natalie Krivanek
Cover design by Ray Lundgren
Manufacturing buyer: John Hall

To my family:
Bill, Craig, and Lynnea Shane
and to all the R.N. students with whom I have worked.

©1983 by Prentice-Hall, Inc., Englewood Cliffs, N.J. 07632

All rights reserved. No part of this book
may be reproduced in any form or
by any means without permission in writing
from the publisher.

Printed in the United States of America

10 9 8 7 6 5 4 3 2 1

ISBN 0-13-779157-7 {PBK}
ISBN 0-13-779165-8

Prentice-Hall International, Inc., *London*
Prentice-Hall of Australia Pty. Limited, *Sydney*
Editora Prentice-Hall do Brasil, Ltda., *Rio de Janeiro*
Prentice-Hall Canada Inc., *Toronto*
Prentice-Hall of India Private Limited, *New Delhi*
Prentice-Hall of Japan, Inc., *Tokyo*
Prentice-Hall of Southeast Asia Pte. Ltd., *Singapore*
Whitehall Books Limited, *Wellington, New Zealand*

Contents

PART IV   UNDERSTANDING YOURSELF AS STUDENT

PART V   TRANSITIONS—UNIVERSAL PHENOMENA

Preface

Returning to School: A Guide for Nurses is a book for nurses who are back in school again, or who are thinking about returning to school. Our intent is to help these nurses succeed in their returning-to-school efforts. After reading this book, the nurse should be able to:

1. Identify several historical trends in the development of educational mobility for nurses;
2. Identify the critical aspects of choosing a particular educational program;
3. Understand the etiology, stages, and treatment of the Returning-to-School Syndrome;
4. Relate role theory, culture shock, future shock, change shock, and role shock to returning-to-school experiences;
5. Utilize an increased knowledge of the academic environment, including goals, values, usual operating procedures, and needed skills as a means of enhancing success as a student;
6. Search for resources interpersonally, within the family or workplace environment, within academia and within the profession, as a means for achieving important educational goals;
7. Explore intrapersonal issues that have an impact upon success in academia, such as adult life stage, management of priorities, organization of multiple roles, ability to manage stress, and ability to utilize assertiveness techniques appropriately;

8. Utilize an understanding of adult learning theories as a means of improving the academic performance;

9. Develop a broader perspective of nursing's strides toward professionalism;

10. Devise strategies for applying the knowledge gained in the nurse-student transitions to other life transitions;

11. Compare and contrast individual returning-to-school experiences and feelings with those of others who may have similar or different backgrounds and histories.

Depending upon where you are in the returning-to-school process, certain parts of this book will become either very important to you, or will be unnecessary. For the nurse who is beginning to explore the possibilities of returning to school, it is most important for you to read *all* of Part I. If you are already enrolled in a program, you can skip Chapter Two. Chapter Three may or may not have relevance for you; skim it for ideas you might profitably use. If you are a nurse who is very knowledgeable about issues in nursing and have a thorough understanding of the history of educational mobility for nurses, and you are already enrolled in a nursing program, you could probably begin with Chapter Four.

Part II contains four related chapters that attempt to answer the questions: How do nurses feel when they return to school? How can a knowledge of these typical feelings help nurses as they return? Chapters 5, 6, and 7 report the findings of a six-year field study done in a representative baccalaureate program that admits both nurses and non-nurse (generic) students. These chapters focus on the *meaning* of returning to school as perceived by the nurse-students. Their written and spoken words are organized in a conceptual framework entitled the Returning-to-School Syndrome (RTSS) that provides a structure for communicating the sometimes pleasant, sometimes painful aspects of returning to school. Chapter 8 reviews some strategies for dealing with the Returning-to-School Syndrome.

Part III continues the advice. Chapter 9 tells you how to make the best use of groups in your school environment, and Chapter 10 gives some concrete information on how to muster your interpersonal strengths when dealing with the stresses of returning to school.

Part IV brings together four chapters that present different aspects of the adult student experience in higher education. Chapter 11 reviews the current literature on adult education theories. This review points up the dearth of basic research on adult learners. We know much more about the surface characteristics of adult learners than we know about how adults learn new roles, or, perhaps more crucial for educationally mobile nurses, how roles are expanded and modified most effectively. Chapter 12 reviews the best known theories in adult development and relates these to returning-to-school issues. Chapter 13 deals with one of the most frightening and intimidating aspects of returning to school: written and clinical testing. The "validation" of a nurse's prior knowledge is becoming a very common entry requirement in the many schools admitting educationally mobile nurses, and such testing is inevitably a part of every educational program at some point. Chapter 14 reports the findings of an important research project that studied a large sample of returning-to-school nurses. This research identified the role expectations held by returning nurses at the time they entered their second nursing program, and how these expectations had changed by the time the nurses left the program.

The theme running through Part V's four chapters is that transitions occur at *every* educational level, to non-nurses as well as nurses. Chapter 15 reports that nurses returning to work, after successfully finishing school, experience changes in roles and in their conception of themselves. Chapters 16, 17 and 18 review transitions experienced at the LPN to ADN level, and at the masters and doctoral levels. Obviously, the content of these programs differs enormously. The role transitions, however, are very similar. Important information is given in Chapters 17 and 18 about choosing graduate programs in nursing so that nurses who are returning to school can do some long-term planning about their educational and career futures. Finally, lest readers become slightly paranoid in thinking that role transitions occur only to nurses, Chapter 19 discusses Returning-to-School Syndrome effects observed in non-nurse adult students who return to college. Transitions are in progress all over every campus—at least in those areas where role changes are occurring.

This book, then, consists of information, advice, theory, and reports that attempt to capture the *actuality* of the returning to school experience of nurses at this time. Commonalities in these experiences transcend personality mixes, curricular practices, or geographic locations. Nurses everywhere grapple with very similar concerns, and our intent is to convey to each reader a sense of how other nurses have felt, coped, and succeeded in their returning to school efforts.

I am very grateful to the RN students with whom I have worked over the past six years. They have proven themselves to be resourceful, resilient, committed, and capable individuals; without their willingness to share their insecurities, sorrows, failures, and anxieties as well as their triumphs, humor, and joy with me, this book would not have been written. I must also acknowledge the professional support and help I have received from my colleagues. They are dedicated educators who have repeatedly demonstrated their concern for their nurse-students.

I must acknowledge the deep debt I owe the New Mexico System for Nursing Articulation Program (SNAP). As a staff member for three years and a close associate for two additional years, my knowledge about educational mobility for nurses was increased a hundredfold. Project Director Mary Jane Ferrell was unfailingly supportive. The project was funded by the W. K. Kellogg Foundation from 1975 through 1980.

The typists who produced the manuscript get a big "Thank You." Donna Southard; Pam Burkhardt; Ginger Beck; and my mother, Berea Carl, did the most.

Finally, I must convey my deep gratitude to the contributors who have shared with us their expertise, viewpoints, and nuggets of advice. They took time out of their very busy professional lives to produce, in a very short amount of time, their contributions. Our gratitude will be their only rewards for this effort, but it is large and sincerely given.

Returning to school is a tremendous adventure for a nurse. It requires a risk-taking personality, careful planning, the gathering of needed resources, training in crucial skills, detailed knowledge of unfamiliar settings, and a commitment to enjoying an activity that demands stretching one's personal capabilities beyond the normal day-to-day limits. Returning to school becomes an investment in one's self. The rewards may be immediate, or they may be years in coming, but—without exception—benefits accrue to those who successfully reach their academic goals. Furthermore, we believe that returning to school can be successfully accomplished by nurses who are well-informed about the process, who are competent in the skills needed in academia, and who are committed to their own development as nurses and as people. We hope this book serves as a useful guide to these nurses.

Donea L. Shane, R.N., M.S.

CONTRIBUTORS

Charlotte Abbink, R.N., M.S.N.
Assistant Professor
University of New Mexico
College of Nursing
Albuquerque, New Mexico

Martha S. Albert, Ph.D.
Management Consultant and Adjunct
Assistant Professor,
Robert O. Anderson
  Schools of Management,
  University of New Mexico

Donna M. Arlton, R.N., M.S., Ed.D.
Dean and Professor
School of Nursing and Gerontology
University of Northern Colorado
Greeley, Colorado

Susan W. Crawford, R.N., Ph.D.
Coordinator, Nursing Mobility
Inver Hills Community College
Inver Grove Heights, Minnesota

Shirley Murphy Curtis, B.S.N., M.S.
Director and Assistant Professor
School of Nursing
University of Denver
Denver, Colorado

Joan V. Dixson, R.N., A.A.N., B.S.N.
Head Nurse, Rehabilitation Unit
St. Joseph Hospital
Albuquerque, New Mexico

Mary Jane Ferrell, R.N., M.S.N
Doctoral Candidate, Secondary
  and Adult Teacher Education
University of New Mexico
Albuquerque, New Mexico

Helen Hamilton, R.N., M.S.N.
Assistant Professor/Retention
  Counselor
University of New Mexico
College of Nursing
Albuquerque, New Mexico

Patricia Grant Higgins, R.N., M.S.N.
Visiting Instructor
University of New Mexico
College of Nursing
Albuquerque, New Mexico

William L. Holzemer, Ph.D.
Assistant Professor
School of Nursing
University of California, San Francisco

Katherine L. Jako, Ph.D.
Associate
Sonoma State University
Rohnert Park, California

Linda A. Kelly, R.N., M.S.
Instructor
Russell Sage School of Nursing
Albany, New York

Patricia Luna, Ed.S.
Formerly Re-entry and Transfer
  Coordinator
Office of School Relations
University of New Mexico
Albuquerque, New Mexico

Judith T. Maurin, R.N., Ph.D.
Associate Professor and Acting Dean
University of New Mexico
College of Nursing
Albuquerque, New Mexico

Myra Moldenhauer, R.N., B.S.N.
Inservice Assistant,
  Post Anesthesia Recovery
St. Joseph Hospital
Albuquerque, New Mexico

Donea L. Carl Shane, R.N., M.S.
Assistant Professor and Coordinator
  for Undergraduate R.N. Students
University of New Mexico
College of Nursing
Albuquerque, New Mexico

Janice Thornburg, R.N., M.S.N.
Instructor, Psychiatric and
   Community Health Nursing
University of New Mexico
College of Nursing
Albuquerque, New Mexico

Karen Bergman Tomajan, R.N., B.S.N.
Department of Nursing Career
   Development
Presbyterian Hospital
Oklahoma City, Oklahoma

Landra White, M.A.
Counselor
Women's Center
University of New Mexico
Albuquerque, New Mexico

PART ONE
AN INTRODUCTION TO EDUCATIONAL MOBILITY FOR NURSES

1

The Evolution of Nursing and Its Impact on You

Donea L. Shane, R.N., M.S.

The semester has started, barely; the week has been quiet for me—a slow easing into [the semester]. Last fall, the extremeness of emotions I felt were great, with much lashing out at the inequities and unfairnesses. Much of that has quelled, softened, and been dispelled by time and experience at the game-of-school.

After dabbling at the prerequisites for one year, I was encouraged very positively [by a faculty member] to apply to the school of nursing. This required some intensive footwork on my part, to finish 16 credit hours, take the challenge tests—and to be bright eyed and eager for the beginning of the fall semester last year. At the same time, I was negotiating school around a 24-hours-per-week work schedule plus single-parenting three children ages 7, 11, and 13 years.

As that first fall semester arrived, I looked forward to the classes—the health assessment class especially—as something I'd enjoy and gain from. Also along with my course load, I brought with me more than my share of guilt over the time pressures, role demands and meeting the needs of others. It was a demanding semester, requiring some major changes in my approach to school, my handling of the children and my ability to be flexible and adaptive.

These were indeed unchartered waters for the former "Super Mom" I had always been. That role ended. In its place came an arrangement of mutual cooperation and habitation. Each child took on and became absolutely responsible for certain tasks. The emphasis switched from my role as mother, to each of us having a role where we mutually exist. We all live together and each of us has become increasingly independent and responsible.

Academically, I had much work and many mental machinations prior to "allowing" myself to be a B student without constant self-flagellation. Recognizing my own limitations, prioritizing my time and then being able to let the

1

rest go came with great difficulty to me. The course work was demanding. At times I felt it was inordinately demeaning and at other times I was certain they were making things far more difficult than they needed to be.

Poor communication between students and faculty sometimes led to major misunderstandings. Yet through it all there were experiences and people who stood out as excellent instructors, supporters and friends.

Where does that leave me this semester? I feel more relaxed about the whole process. It *will* all get done. My anxiety runs far lower. The [challenge] was a positive experience. I feel ready to move on, prepared for some of the dips that certainly are ahead—but more importantly, ready to give a bit, aware of the need for flexibility and not obsessed with fighting the system.

R.N., mid-thirties,
from a diary

This excerpt from a diary kept by a nurse who recently returned to school illustrates the exceedingly complex nature of this activity. The process of returning to school can be mystifying, infuriating, frightening, and exhausting, as well as professionally stimulating, personally growth enhancing, and fun. We believe it is always worthwhile. Most nurses could use some help.

The help in this book is organized around providing information and advice. The information given is factually and theoretically based. The advice, of course, is the opinion of the author. These opinions have been formulated after working for years with nurses who have returned to school. We assume that you, the reader of this book, are a nurse who is engaged in the returning-to-school process. We want to help you succeed in reaching your educational goal because we believe that increasing the educational attainments of today's nurses is important to the profession of nursing. Education will prepare the nursing leaders, thinkers, researchers, and innovators the profession must have to continue to provide high-quality service to society. Individuals always benefit from further education, we believe. The educational process fosters positive changes in skills, thinking abilities, and knowledge, as well as introducing one to an exciting and unique social setting. Career paths and lifestyles may change dramatically following the pursuit of additional education. The noble goal of self-actualization—becoming all that you can be—is facilitated by the educational process in many instances. Returning to school can be the beginning of important changes in your life, and the educational goals that you set for yourself are important.

TERMINOLOGY

We have tried to keep the use of jargon to a minimum, but it is important that we define a few key words and phrases that appear repeatedly in this text.

Educationally mobile nurse is a phrase used to describe the person who is a nurse (an L.P.N. or an R.N. of any educational background) who is enrolled or seeking enrollment in an institution of higher education. Educationally mobile nurses come in two sexes; we have varied the use of pronouns in the text so that either "he" or "she" can refer to the nurse. By definition, the educationally mobile person is already a *nurse*. Thus current enrollment is at least the second entry to an educational program; it may be the third, fourth, or fifth in fact. Furthermore, the clear bias in this book (we may just as well admit this at the outset) is that the nurse is enrolling in a legitimate *nursing* program, rather than in a nonnursing major or a program that recruits nurses but teaches nothing about nursing. Educationally mobile nurses are energetic, special people. We want to help them as much as we can, because they bring a unique and valuable perspective to nursing. The term "mobilist" is a synonym for the "educationally mobile nurse."

Career mobility is a general term usually used to designate a "movement from any one level to another in an occupational field. As such it may refer to a range from the lowest to the highest levels of preparation. It usually refers to movement in an upward direction, although it also may designate lateral mobility" (Lenburg, 1975, p. 26). We have used the term "career mobility" infrequently in this book because our focus is primarily on the educational level, not on the occupational level. However, in the general nursing literature, there appears to be fuzziness and overlap in the use of the terms "career mobility" and "educational mobility."

School, as in "Returning to School: A Guide for Nurses," refers to any organized program of learning located in a legitimate institution that has as a major function the conveying of knowledge, skills, and attitudes to enrollees. This could be an associate degree in nursing program or a hospital diploma school that admits Licensed Practical Nurses (L.P.N.s or L.V.N.s), a baccalaureate program in nursing (the usual degree conferred for completing this program is a Bachelor of Science in Nursing, B.S.N.), or a program offering a master's or doctorate.

Higher education is a phrase that broadly denotes programs located in colleges or universities. It is sometimes distinguished from *vocational education*, a phrase used to identify programs that focus on developing job skills. Higher education is always more advanced than high school. Vocational education may occur in high schools or following high school and is more narrowly focused than higher education, which is always concerned with the development of the total individual beyond job-related skills.

The *mainstream of higher education* is a phrase repeatedly heard in nursing. "Mainstream" educational programs occur in colleges or universities, such as A.D.N. and B.S.N. programs. In nursing, nonmainstream programs occur in hospital diploma schools of nursing. Hospital diploma schools are defined as being outside the mainstream of higher education because they are funded differently and are not accredited by the same six regional accrediting associations that accredit universities (although some hospital schools of nursing are moving to become members of these accrediting groups.) Also, hospitals obviously have more functions than the education of students; they are multipurpose institutions.

The nonmainstream status of hospital diploma schools has a major impact on educationally mobile nurses moving from a hospital diploma school background into a mainstream school. Mainstream schools have established agreements about how they will accept transfer credits from each other; these policies define the meaning of "college credit" and represent the standards for higher education. These policies govern all departments, not just the nursing schools, and essentially the policies prohibit transferring credits earned in a nonmainstream setting into a mainstream school. An additional problem is that nonmainstream schools may not issue "credit" per se or adhere to an academic calendar, thereby increasing the chances that no transferability can occur. Nursing is not the only profession that has both mainstream and nonmainstream educational programs, but nursing seems to have more of them and to have sustained them longer into the twentieth century than other groups. Nursing will be in the mainstream of higher education when all nursing schools award academic credit, give standard academic degrees, and are eligible to be members of the higher education regional accrediting associations.

An *academic degree* is a rank, symbolized by initials placed after your name, awarded by a college or university for completing a required course of study. Associate degrees are given after completing two years of schooling, usually in a junior college or a community college; baccalaureate degrees are given after completing four years of school. "Bachelor's degree" and "baccalaureate degree" are synonymous. Master's degrees are conferred upon people after they have completed one or two years of college work beyond a baccalaureate, and doctoral degrees usually require four to five years beyond the baccalaureate. Hospital diplomas are not considered academic degrees because they are not conferred by a college or university. This is not, however, a judgment on the worth of a hospital diploma education, nor on the value and skill that diploma school graduates bring to health care. It is simply an outcome of the educational establishment's policies; these policies apply to all disciplines for which people are educated, not just nursing.

Academia is a word derived from the Greek place name Academe, the grove of olive trees near ancient Athens where Plato taught. We use it now to denote colleges and universities that are involved in scholarly work and in which the generation and transmission of knowledge is the focal activity.

The words *"college"* and *"university"* are used interchangeably, although there is a slight technical difference. Universities offer the highest degrees (the doctoral level) and usually contain more than one college that offer degree programs. *Colleges*, which are stand-alone institutions, usually do not offer any degree beyond the master's, and some go only to the baccalaureate level. Universities are usually much larger than colleges. "Junior college" and "community college" are used interchangeably and generally denote two-year schools that offer the associate degree.

NURSING IS EVOLVING

Imagine for a moment that *nursing* (the people who have been or who are now nurses, plus all the writings, events, meetings, pronouncements, organizations, and work done in the name of nursing) can be viewed as an entity with a life of its own; like all living things, it is developing, evolving, and changing. Nursing right now is obviously in a painful period, developmentally, and we know that most developmental crises involve anxiety, tension, conflict, and ambiguity. The transition that nursing is now experiencing can be viewed as the culmination of a number of streams of evolutionary change, all influenced by the environment in which nursing exists in this country. Probably the decision to return to school is made by many nurses because they have personally felt some of the tensions arising out of nursing's current transitional state. Since you may be one of these nurses, it is important that you understand the historical influences that are affecting you at this time.

However, this is not a history text. We will briefly sketch a few of the important developments in nursing, choosing those that appear to have the most impact upon educationally mobile nurses. You may use this very brief discussion as a guide to further investigation of those factors in nursing's evolution that intrigue you.

Major developments in nursing have been as follows:

1. The emergence of modern nursing from a military tradition.
2. The professionalization of nursing.
3. The emergence of diverse educational paths to registered nursing.
4. The Credentialing Study's recommendations for reform.
5. Changes in nursing's scope of practice and method of delivery.

The Florence Nightingale type of schools, transplanted from England to the United States, Canada, and northern Europe, were imperfect copies of the original Nightingale school located at St. Thomas's Hospital in London. Nightingale had established a separately endowed and autonomously administered school; the copies in the United States were supported and thus controlled by local hospitals and their boards of directors. Being educated in hospital schools of nursing was immensely better than having no training at all; but from the very beginning of nursing in this country, the underlying reason for operating a school of nursing was to ensure a supply of well-socialized, highly skilled workers for a particular hospital. Intellectual growth, broad knowledge in the humanities and sciences, or any of the other educational goals of the time were never the primary mission of a hospital school of nursing.

Because there was a dramatic rise in the number of hospitals from the late 1880s to the 1900s, the number of training schools for nurses also rose rapidly. In 1872 only four schools of nursing had opened in the United States, but by 1902 there were 492 in existence (Kalisch and Kalisch, 1978, p. 134). The quality of these schools varied greatly; no formal standards had been promulgated to define who should be admitted to schools of nursing, what sort of curriculum should be followed, or what credentials teachers should have.

Florence Nightingale was influential in the reorganization of the British army medical service; her first school of nursing reflected this military influence, as did the copies in the United States. Like good foot soldiers, good nurses were obedient and strictly disciplined with an expectation that improper behavior would be punished. They were socialized into a ranking system in which they were near the bottom. They had to be willing to sacrifice their health and their lives for their calling. Good soldiers and good nurses did not question their superiors, did not complain about long hours in the field, and did not expect handsome pay or plush living quarters. Good soldiers and good nurses were not expected to think through unusual problems or to suggest strategies; they were taught to stay alert, sound an alarm when the situation warranted, and then to follow the orders given by their superiors. Good soldiers and good nurses wore their uniforms proudly, knew their duties well, and always did what had to be done.

Officers in the military, of course, were usually educated gentlemen who assumed their positions only after they had completed a basic university education or had graduated from a military academy that was a specialized university. Even today the enlisted ranks in the military are filled with people who have less than a college education. Movement into the officer corps without a college education is difficult; once in the enlisted ranks, a person is rewarded for meritorious service by moving up the enlisted ranks, not by being placed into the officer corps. Those people in the military who make the policies, lead the troops, and assume responsibility for the decisions and outcomes of activities are always college educated.

Several studies of nursing have noted the lack of a cadre of "officer-level" nurses, those nurses who would be broadly educated, sophisticated, and capable of assuming responsibility for long-range outcomes. The Goldmark Report, published in 1923 and entitled "Nursing and Nursing Education in the United States," emphasized the importance of establishing university schools of nursing in order to train nursing leaders (Kalisch and Kalisch, 1978, p. 334). In 1948, Esther Lucille Brown authored "Nursing for the Future." This report spurred efforts to study the quality of schools of nursing in the country. Brown noted that many hospitals still operated schools of nursing in order to avail themselves of the services of student nurses. She recommended that "effort be directed to building basic schools of nursing in universities and colleges, comparable in number to existing medical schools, that are sound in organizational and financial structure, adequate in facilities and faculty, and well distributed to serve the needs of the entire country" (Brown, 1948, pp. 48, 178). She recommended two levels of practice: the college-educated professional and the licensed practical nurse. In 1950, the National Committee for the Improvement of Nursing Services published a report entitled "Nursing Schools at the Mid-Century." They noted the startling fact that, of the 10,000 instructors teaching in American schools of nursing, 45 percent had no academic degree (West and Hawkins, 1950). The Committee on the Function of Nursing chaired by Eli Ginzberg (1948) defended the need for two levels of nursing practice.

In 1963, the Consultant Group on Nursing, appointed by the Surgeon General of the U.S. Public Health Service, released a report entitled "Toward Quality in Nursing: Needs and Goals." This report recommended that nursing education be studied in relation to the responsibilities and skill levels required for high-quality patient care, and suggested that a position paper on nursing education from the professional association would be a helpful resource. In response, "A Position Paper on Educational Preparation for Nurse Practitioners and Assistants to Nurses" was published by the American Nurses Association (ANA) in 1965.

The ANA position paper made these points:

1. The education for all those who are licensed to practice nursing should take place in institutions of higher education.

2. Minimum preparation for beginning professional nursing practice

at the present time should be baccalaureate education in nursing.

3. Minimum preparation for beginning technical nursing practice at the present time should be the associate degree education in nursing.

4. Education for assistants in the health-care occupations should be short, intensive preservice programs in vocational education institutions rather than on-the-job training programs.

Despite the fact that "two-level" proposals had been recommended for nearly forty years, publication of the ANA position paper fell like a bombshell dropped on an unsuspecting population. Some nurses felt that their professional organization had labeled them "unprofessional" if they did not have a baccalaureate degree. Nearly everyone connected with hospital schools of nursing could find some reason to be furious. Although diploma schools were the dominant form of nursing education at the time, the position paper did not support their continued existence, but suggested that diploma schools participate instead with colleges and universities in the planning of baccalaureate programs or A.D.N. programs. This suggestion caused enormous dismay among hospital administrators, diploma nursing educators, alumni of nursing schools, and enrolled students. Since 78 percent of the nurses in practice as of 1965 were graduates of diploma programs, the pool of disgruntled constituents was large (ANA, 1966).

The ANA has continued to maintain the position that there should be two levels of nursing in this country. In spite of a dramatic decline in membership (a reported 19 percent decline between 1975 and 1980) and a decline in the percentage of practicing nurses who are members (41 percent in 1958 down to 13 percent in 1980), and despite an ANA-sponsored study which showed that the "entry into practice" issue was the most significant issue confronting the state nurses associations (ANA, 1981), no change in the position has occurred. The explanation for this surely lies in the perceived "moral integrity" of the position paper in terms of its importance to the professionalization of nursing, and a recognition that the professional society (ANA) is the appropriate body to raise educational standards in nursing.

Robert K. Merton, a well-known contemporary sociologist, served as a consultant sociologist to the ANA. His writings on the function of the professional association have been influential in setting the course of the ANA's stands and are worth noting here. In a 1958 article, he explicates the functions of the professional association as follows:

> The foremost obligation of the association is to set rigorous standards
> for the profession and to help enforce them: standards for the quality of per-

sonnel to be recruited into the profession; standards for the training and education of the recruits; standards for professional practice; and standards for research designed to enlarge the knowledge on which the work of the profession rests . . . .

The professional association is a kind of organizational gadfly, stinging the profession into new and more demanding formulations of purpose. It must therefore be prepared to become a target for hostile criticism from those members of the profession who find themselves or feel themselves disadvantaged by the continuing forward thrust toward raising the standards of the profession . . . . At any time in the history of a profession, its members are variously trained and variously competent, since they have entered the field at different times. The less highly trained, naturally enough, look with some displeasure, if not despair, at the rising standards of qualifications for professional practice.

Professionalization of Nursing

Gamer (1979) notes that, while nursing in its early days was involved in the struggle to obtain licensure, improve schools, and secure reasonable wages and better working conditions, it was united in its understanding that professionalism was defined as completing a training program, being a respectable person, taking pride in one's skills, and being committed to ethical principles. Nurses adapted to a system that gave them responsibility without authority to make decisions about the nursing care given to patients. Other thinkers and writers on the professionalization of nursing have compared nursing to Flexner's (1910) classic characteristics of a profession: a profession is basically intellectual with great personal responsibility; it is based on lengthy education that conveys a unique body of knowledge; it is practical; its techniques can be taught; it is strongly organized internally; and it is motivated by altruism. Etzioni (1969) differentiated between the "full-fledged" professions and the "semi-professions." As one criterion, he used five years or more of education as the dividing line between the two. Nursing, of course, he grouped with the "semi-professions."

Jacox (1978) identifies three major criteria for a profession: (1) a long period of specialized education, (2) a service orientation, and (3) autonomy, which means that members of the profession are self-regulating and have control of their functions in the work setting. Nursing has a long history of commitment to service. The problems in achieving professional status have crystallized around two major issues: the educational process that leads to professional performance and the degree of control nurses have over their practice. Gamer (1979) makes the point that this focus on autonomy and education as the route to professionalism includes an abandoning of the stance that nurses possess unique clinical competencies. These unique competencies (if such exist) could serve as a platform for convincing society that nursing is an essential service and unquestionably a profession.

Perhaps nursing has spent such tremendous amounts of energy and time on attempting to reform its educational programs because education is the arena most under the control of nursing and, therefore, most amenable to change. Certainly, gaining complete autonomy over nursing practice in most bureaucratic settings seems a distant goal: Both hospital administration and physicians' control over nursing practice mitigate against autonomy for the practicing staff nurse. The movements toward unionization of nursing services can be interpreted as a step in this direction, although as yet there is little evidence that individual nurses gain more control of their practice under union contracts.

The collaborative practice of physicians and nurses has been tested in four hospitals, with the encouraging results that this joint responsibility for patient-care decision making resulted in improved quality of care and in the satisfaction of both nurses and physicians with their practice (National Commission on Nursing, 1981, p. 11). The truly collaborative, cooperative, equal-but-different relationship between physicians and nurses in the care of their clients has not, however, moved beyond the experimental stage in this country. Indeed, most state laws support the physician's orders as the legitimate source of nursing activities. Thus it appears that, for the near future, nurses will continue to rely upon their skills at playing "the doctor–nurse game" in order to vicariously control their practice decisions. (The "doctor–nurse game," is described by Stein, 1967, as a transactional neurosis in which the doctor must depend upon the nurse for both information and recommendations for patient treatment in particular situations; the nurse supplies these recommendations in such a manner that they appear to be initiated by the physician.)

Should Nursing Professionalize?

This is a "values" question that perhaps is not asked publicly often enough. Nursing leaders and nursing educators usually *assume* that continuing to fight the good fight for the professionalization of nursing is something that all nurses automatically want. There is evidence, however, that substantial numbers of nurses (1) do not understand the issues of professionalization, and thus participate inappropriately in professionalizing movements, (2) do not want nursing to change from the current status quo, and thereby continue to reinforce the present semiprofessional state of nursing, and (3) do not wish to gain the responsibilities that accompany belonging to a professionalized work force and therefore actively work to defeat current professionalization efforts. The pieces of evidence we offer for this argument are (1) the lack of a well-supported professional society in nursing, (2) the active involvement of nurses in defeating efforts to upgrade nursing education standards, and (3) the reluctance of some nurses to function autonomously (and thus accept direct responsibility for client outcomes) when given the opportunity to do so.

What would happen if all the professionalization efforts were stopped tomorrow? What if we did away with the professional society (the American Nurses Association), closed all the nursing schools above the level of the diploma or associate degree, stopped the practitioner movement, abandoned our efforts to gain control of our nursing practices, stopped all the research being done by nurses, and agreed among ourselves that we would be content with practicing a vocation? The vocation of nursing would probably be hospital-based; the role taught in nursing schools would be exceedingly reality based, with little time spent on "superfluous" knowledge. Nurses would not need to be broadly educated because they would be under the control of hospital policies and the direction of physicians. There would be no need to train researchers, educators, or even leaders because other professions would perform those services, if they were needed at all.

Forces both within and outside nursing seem to be voting on the side of maintaining nursing as a vocation. It is quite possible that our inabilities to gain consensus on whether (or how) the professionalization of nursing should proceed will mean that key decisions will be made *for* us, not *by* us.

Would nursing be able to attract qualified newcomers if it remained a vocation? Would salaries continue to rise if we gave up our claims to professionalization? Would the nursing shortage be relieved? Would patient care be improved? Would health-care costs rise or decline? Would nursing be able to respond to changing health-care needs? Would the public be better served by a *vocation* of nursing rather than a *profession* of nursing? Does society need aspects of both?

We ask these questions to stimulate your thinking on these points. Educationally mobile nurses are in key positions to understand the ramifications of nursing's vocational and/or professional future; keep these questions in mind as you proceed through school. It is important that all of us clarify our values on the professionalization of nursing.

Emergence of Diverse Educational Pathways to Nursing

Hospital diploma schools of nursing were the original and, until very recently, the most numerous type of nursing school in this country. We have seen how they arose from the Nightingale tradition and rapidly spread throughout the United States. There seems to be general agreement that the strengths of hospital diploma school nursing education lie in the emphasis upon technical proficiency, the thorough socialization processes that occur, the large amount of hospital clinical experience obtained by the student, and the reality orientation of the role presented to the student. The number of hospital schools has been declining steadily over the past three decades. This represents a "weeding-out" process; the schools that remain are usually accredited by the National League for Nursing (NLN) (91 percent of diploma schools were accredited in 1977), with stable faculty, curricula, and good-quality facilities (NLN, 1978).

Associate degree nursing schools grew out of a five-year (1952–1957) pilot project that studied the feasibility of two-year nursing programs placed within junior or community colleges. Mildred Montag, the director of the pilot project, worked with seven community colleges to develop and evaluate the pilot programs. The evaluation of the original pilot project schools was positive, showing that nurses could function effectively in hospital settings and could successfully pass state board examinations (91.7 percent of the pilot study graduates passed the exams on the first attempt).

Associate degree nursing education grew out of the vocational education movement in American education (Safier, 1977, p. 219) and the belief that nursing functions could be differentiated into technical and professional roles (Montag, 1980). The original intent included the development of (1) a knowledge base dealing primarily with the technical tasks of nursing, (2) a strong social consciousness, (3) a role in which the graduate was responsible for recognizing problems of a recurring predictable nature and for planning, implementing, and evaluating daily assignments, and (4) a nursing role in which the graduate worked under the supervision of the professional nurse (Kohnke, 1973, p. 1572). Recently, Bullough (1979) noted that the A.D.N. graduate "has emerged as the basic hospital nurse." The rise in the number of associate degree graduates in nursing has been phenomenal. In 1953, 260 people graduated from all the A.D.N. programs in the country. In 1976, the number of A.D.N. graduates was 35,094, which established this form of nursing education as the dominant one today (Kalisch and Kalisch, 1978, p. 652). The dominance of A.D.N. education was neither planned for nor predicted by the nursing establishment; it can be viewed as parallel to the growth of junior colleges in this country.

University schools of nursing that offer the baccalaureate degree in nursing have existed since the opening of the University of Minnesota School of Nursing in 1909. During the early years, most university schools of nursing were in reality diploma schools that added a year or two of college work, so the graduate received both a diploma and a degree (Kalisch and Kalisch, 1978, p. 337). The first autonomous collegiate school of nursing was established at Yale, with Annie Goodrich as its dean; but the admission standards were later elevated to requiring a baccalaureate degree as the entry credential, and a Master of Nursing degree was awarded to its graduates (Kalisch and Kalisch, 1978, p. 339). That program has remained unique; the standard for collegiate education for nurses is the baccalaureate degree.

Through the years, it has been the hope of most leaders in nursing that university schools of nursing would produce graduates who would (1) be capable of performing scientifically based nursing care in a manner superior to that of performing technical tasks under close supervision, (2) be as well educated (and thus as sophisticated, socially equal, and as well paid) as other college graduates, (3) be actively committed to the professionalization of nursing, and (4) be capable of and prepared for further education at the master's and doctoral levels.

Both the number of baccalaureate programs and the number of graduates from those programs have risen steadily but not dramatically over the past three decades. In 1953, 2,171 people graduated from B.S.N. programs; in 1976, 22,678 graduated (Kalisch and Kalisch, 1978). This steady growth pattern, contrasted to the enormous growth in associate degree programs, is probably a function of the larger expense in terms of both faculty and tuition for four-year programs, the reluctance of some university faculties to acknowledge the legitimacy of nursing as an academic discipline, the dearth of qualified nurse faculty members, and the comparatively minor commitment to nursing education by university officials, as contrasted to the vigorous commitment demonstrated by the administrators of junior and community colleges.

Educational Mobility in Nursing

When there was only one form of nursing education in this country, there was no educational mobility, obviously. Only after two routes to registered nursing had been established (diploma plus university schools) did educational mobility for nurses become an issue. We can identify three eras in nursing educational mobility: (1) the years from the establishment of a second form of nursing education (1909) to the time in 1960 when the NLN Baccalaureate and Higher Degree Council made a key policy decision regarding how registered nurses should be handled within university settings; (2) the years between 1960 and 1972, when established schools utilized the NLN policies to accommodate nurses returning to school; and (3) from 1972, the date when the first upper-division nursing programs for registered nurses only were established, to the present.

The early years, 1909 to 1960, were a time of diversity. Registered nurses who applied to a university program could be asked to start at the beginning of the freshman year and complete everything, including the nursing, in order to earn the baccalaureate degree. Most schools required R.N.s to complete only the general education courses. There was wide variation in the amount of credit awarded for completion of the diploma program, and the techniques for determining which credits, and how many, were to be awarded for the diploma also varied (Conley, 1973, p. 573). The number of R.N.s completing university programs was relatively small, but included many of nursing's present leaders. Many schools offered specialized programs in nursing education or nursing administration at the baccalaureate level for registered nurses.

The middle era in nursing educational mobility, from 1960 to 1972, was inaugurated when the NLN adopted a policy for baccalaureate programs that was based on the consensus that there should be a single program in nursing leading to a baccalaureate degree, not one for generic students and another for the registered nurses who entered a school. As Conley (1973, p. 573) reports, NLN Baccalaureate and Higher Degree Council members agreed that, since nursing was the educational major, some upper-division courses in nursing should be required of all students. Furthermore, since the baccalaureate program in nursing prepares the general practitioner, it was deemed inappropriate to continue programs that prepared R.N.s for teaching and administration at the baccalaureate level. "Blanket" credit for diploma nursing courses was outlawed. Schools moved to implement this policy change during the years that associate degree schools were proliferating and graduates were seeking entry to university baccalaureate programs; these changes also were implemented during the years when the ANA Position Paper (1965) was causing much concern and consternation among diploma and A.D.N. nurses. Lenburg (1975, p. 28) notes that

> Although the educators who accepted the statement [that there could be only a single program in nursing leading to the baccalaureate degree] may have felt that the cause of "quality" education had been served, there is little wonder that R.N.s seeking career mobility continued to raise cries of frustration and anguish with an insensitive and unresponsive system. The profession may have taken a step forward, but it did little to reconcile the dilemma of the motivated and able R.N.

By 1970, the "cries of frustration and anguish" had stimulated the National League for Nursing's board of directors to endorse the development and implementation of "open curriculum practices" in accredited schools of nursing. A privately funded Open Curriculum Project was initiated by the NLN in 1971 (Lenburg and Johnson, 1974) to survey educational mobility practices in all nursing schools in the country, to publish a directory of schools with open-curriculum practices already in place, and to study selected pilot project programs with the ultimate goal of preparing national guidelines for open-curriculum approaches (Lenburg, 1975, pp. 44–45). The open-curriculum survey found that 15,000 students with past education or experience in nursing or other allied health occupations were enrolled in programs at that time. Patterns of educational mobility were evident: L.P.N.s were twice as likely to gain advanced placement into associate degree programs than into baccalaureate programs; between 76 and 79 percent of diploma, associate degree, and baccalaureate programs offered advanced placement opportunities to educationally mobile applicants; and utilization of examinations for evaluation of placement was by far the most dominant practice (Johnson, 1975, p. 55). This survey also identified the time and effort payoffs to students for open-curriculum practices. Eighty-six percent of the baccalaureate schools reported practices that reduced the length of the program; 61 percent of the diploma schools and 60 percent of the associate degree schools also reported practices that reduced the length of time L.P.N.s spent in the registered nurse educational program (Johnson, 1975, p. 57).

Thus the middle era of educational mobility for nurses was a time that included both an initial narrowing of opportunities for interested nurses and a later period in which increased attention was given to the special needs of this important group of potential nursing students.

The present era, which we have identified as beginning in 1972 with the establishment of the first upper-division programs for R.N.s only, has seen the development and growth of a number of different kinds of nursing education programs intended to meet the needs of educationally mobile nurses.

Nursing programs designed expressly for educationally mobile registered nurses may have a variety of names: second step, upper two, two plus two, B.R.N. programs, career ladder, or B.S.N.-R.N. are some of the more common designations. These programs consist of upper-division majors in nursing and are usually located in institutions that do not have a generic nursing program. Vaughn (1980) reports that between 1975 and 1979 this type of program grew in number from 50 to 99. During the same period, enrollments doubled, from about 5,000 to over 10,600. Between the fall of 1971 when one of the first such programs was established at Sonoma State College in California, to the NLN report in 1979, nearly 100 baccalaureate programs designed specifically for R.N.s had been established. This growth in programs (again unplanned for and not predicted by the nursing establishment) echoes the rapid growth of associate degree schools in the 1960s.

One dysfunction resulting from such rapid growth has been difficulty in applying the existing accreditation criteria to what are essentially nontraditional approaches to baccalaureate nursing education. The NLN's criteria for accreditation include some aspects that are by definition impossible (or nearly so) for programs that are committed to building professional performance upon a lower-division nursing base. Studies of the accreditation criteria have been undertaken, and some operational changes have been implemented in an effort to accommodate to the changing character of baccalaureate nursing education. However, by 1981 less than a quarter of the upper-division R.N.-only programs had been NLN accredited.

During the period of 1975 to 1979, the number of registered nurses enrolled in more traditional baccalaureate programs that admit generic students increased dramatically also, from 10,800 to 17,300. By 1979, 429 schools of nursing in the country admitted registered nurses; 28,033 R.N.s were enrolled in such programs (Vaughn, 1980).

The Carnegie Commission on the Future of Higher Education conducted a series of studies that highlighted the general public's rather jaundiced view of higher education during the late 1960s. In their report, the commission recommended that

> professions, wherever possible, create alternate routes of entry other than full-time college attendance, and reduce the number of narrow, one-level professions which do not afford opportunities for advancement . . . a degree (or other form of credit) should be made available to students at least every two years in their careers. (Carnegie Commission, 1971)

That nursing has in place aspects of such a system should be a source of pride to us. Over the past century, it is evident that nursing education has been responsive to changes in society, educational trends, and the needs of the profession.

However, it would be insane to suggest that our current system is even remotely rational. At present in this country one can become a registered nurse by attending a two-, three-, four-, five- or seven-year program. One can enter a basic educational program that will qualify one for taking the state board registered nurse licensure exam by completing an associate degree, a hospital diploma, a baccalaureate degree, a master's degree, or a doctorate. We can trace the social forces that facilitated the development of each of these routes toward the registered nurse licensure, and we can defend their concurrent existence as a part of the evolution of nursing in this country. The key question, however, is if these multiple routes to registered nurse licensure are supportable simply because they presently exist. Other questions nag: Are these programs identical? Are the graduates similar in competency? Why is there such wide variation in the time spent in school?

Nursing's educational system is clearly divergent from the general plan that other professions and disciplines in this country follow for their educational pathways to practice. In other professional or semiprofessional fields, the associate degree is reserved for two-year pre-professional technician programs. A good example of this is the engineering associate degree, which typically focuses on the technical skills necessary to perform some specialized function in a particular industry under the direction of professional engineers. In most fields, the baccalaureate degree is the first professional degree, or is required as entry into the master's or doctoral program, which becomes the first professional degree. The baccalaureate degree may serve as the liberal arts portion of the professional's education. In other fields, the master's programs prepare the practicing experts in the field, and doctoral programs prepare the researchers, theoreticians, and master teachers. Professional certificate programs, parallel to nursing's post high school hospital diploma, do not exist in other professions in this country. However, parallels do exist in vocational areas (for example, beauty culture). Because of the unique nature of nursing's pluralistic system, few of nursing's many publics—clients, laypersons, legislators, interested observers, university administrators, hospital administrators, other nurse employers—understand the present system or the vigor with which the current status quo has been defended by concerned nurses.

The Credentialing Study: Recommendations for Reform

Following extensive public hearings and study of the literature, the National Commission on Nursing (1981, p. 47) noted that

> In the current climate of economic constraint, and of decreasing graduations from nursing programs, the viability of the current pluralistic system of nursing education was questioned.... Nursing ... was challenged ... to rationalize its systems of education and practice.

Probably the major effort made recently to rationally study the current chaotic situation in nursing is the work commissioned by the ANA, which resulted in "The Study of Credentialing in Nursing: A New Approach" (1979). This study, conducted by a group of nurses and nonnurses with consultation from a large number of related organizations, begins by clarifying definitions. *Licensure*, awarded by the government, is defined as a protection for the public and is a permit to engage in certain practices. It prohibits others from practicing and uses established standards for evaluation of the eligibility for initial licensure and for the renewal of licensure. Licensure should be reserved for only the professionals in the field, who are accountable for the entire scope of practice. In contrast, *registration* is defined as a listing in an official roster that is maintained by either a governmental or nongovernmental agency and that enables the registered person to use a particular title, attests that certain minimum qualifications have been met and maintained, and is appropriate for use for nurses who are well qualified for "specified functions" in nursing, but are not accountable for the full scope of nursing practice. *Certification* is used to indicate that a licensed professional has met the specifications set by the professional society for entry into *specialty practice*. *Academic degrees* were not defined as a credentialing mechanism, but the Study Committee took the position that the professional society (ANA) should establish the minimal educational degree required for licensure at the entry level. The Study Committee recognized the difficulty many nurses experience in moving from one program to another and recommended that "educational programs should encourage the achievement of the highest aspirations of individuals insofar as they are consonant with their abilities, and should remove artificial barriers to this attainment" (p. 84). The study recommended that a national nursing credentialing center be established to further study and, someday, conduct credentialing in nursing.

Taking these definitions and using our imaginations a little to fill in the details, we suggest that the following scenario is compatible with the credentialing study recommendations.

Registered nurses, graduates of associate degree in nursing programs, would be registered by either state boards of nursing or the national credentialing center. They would be well qualified for performing specified functions (for example, bedside nursing) in hospital settings only (a limited scope of practice). They would probably take a registration competency exam very similar to the present R.N. state board examination (NCLEX-RN), since this current exam tests primarily for minimum competence to practice nursing in the acute-care setting. This group of nurses would not be eligible for certification for specialty practice, but members could return to school to earn the next academic degree, and thus be eligible for the next higher credential in nursing. Their functions, capabilities, and career paths would be similar to today's staff nurse.

Professional licensed nurses, graduates of baccalaureate degree in nursing programs, would be licensed by state boards of nursing after taking a *different* exam than now exists. (The present examination does not test for competency or safety in all areas of nursing practice; for example, it does not test knowledge or safety in the areas of community health nursing, health promotion and maintenance, or in primary care.) These graduates would be accountable and eligible for any beginning professional position in nursing, either in or out of hospital settings. They would be eligible for entry into master's programs in nursing.

Specialty practice in nursing would be taught in master's programs. After a nurse had earned a M.S.N. in a particular clinical specialty (midwifery, any of the practitioner areas, or community health, for example) the nurse would be eligible to attempt the certification exam.

the range of positions for which one is qualified (in hospitals, community health agencies, private practice, clinics, and the like). In its analysis following extensive hearings on nursing practice and nursing education, the National Commission on Nursing (1981, p. 53) noted that

> In the professions that serve patients there frequently is the perception that new graduates lack the ability immediately to perform successfully in the practice setting. Accordingly, there is the perception that new nursing graduates are not prepared immediately to function as professionals in the practice settings. Differences within and among the three basic nursing education programs and lack of differentiation in the employment of the graduates of the three programs—associate degree, diploma, and baccalaureate—lead to misutilization and often underutilization of registered nurses and confusion and conflict between education and practice.

Current examples of the *misutilization* of new graduates include (1) hiring new graduates as head nurses or charge nurses and (2) using nurses proficient in the primary nursing mode in the functional task assignment model. Two examples of the *underutilization* of new graduates are (1) providing no opportunities for new graduates to utilize their skills in physical assessment, taking nursing histories, or performing thorough intake interviews and (2) providing no opportunities for new graduates to utilize their skills in planning continuous care into the home setting. The Commission on Nursing makes the following recommendation: "Appropriate utilization of nurses should be related to the competency obtained in the educational program. There must be common understanding and recognition of the different levels of competence from the different programs" (National Commission on Nursing, 1981, p. 54).

Just what are these "different levels of competency?" McQuaid and Kane (1979) report a review of differences on state board examinations by the graduates of associate degree, diploma, and baccalaureate programs. A major finding was that there was more variability *within* each type of program than *among* the three types. When the total questions were sorted into ten categories, baccalaureate graduates scored highest on five: accountability for practice, social and behavioral sciences, mental health, human relations, and causes of diseases. Diploma graduates scored highest in natural sciences, physical health, manifestations of diseases, theory of medical and nursing care, and nursing measures. Associate degree graduates' category scores were positively correlated with the ranking of diploma graduates, but not with baccalaureate graduates. These findings indicated to the authors that differences were found in nurses' competencies: associate degree and diploma school graduates competencies were similar, but differed from the competencies of baccalaureate graduates.

Aydelotte (1978) identifies these differences in nursing function. The associate degree graduate functions in settings where "the clinical nursing requirements for service have been well identified, well programmed, and where the data with which she must deal are circumscribed and specific. She can function where policies, procedures, and decisions are programmed, or where she will have direct access to someone who can assist her" (p. 355). Aydelotte notes that the baccalaureate graduate cannot be used purely for bedside care, since society cannot afford to pay professionals for something that paraprofessionals can do as well. She suggests that the baccalaureate graduate employed in the hospital setting may be best utilized as a beginning nurse clinician in a specific field, where she will function "in meeting special needs of patients, in planning programs for patients and nursing staff, and in evaluating effectiveness of care" (p. 357). This suggestion represents a departure from the current emphasis upon producing a baccalaureate graduate who is a beginning generalist in all areas of nursing, both in and outside of hospital settings. The graduate of a master's program in nursing functions where knowledge is being developed (it is hoped that master's-prepared nurses will contribute to the development of nursing's knowledge base), where no procedures have been developed as yet, where the graduate is responsible for making decisions when data are unclear or not yet available, and in situations calling for leadership, accountability, and flexible creative approaches to problem solving. In general, this schema is consistent with the Minimum Behavioral Expectations of New Graduates from New Mexico Schools of Nursing (Ferrell, 1979). Nursing workers with the least education are expected to perform the most concrete, structured, and clearly controlled aspects of nursing; nursing workers who have had more education are expected to perform less structured, more ambiguous, and therefore less controlled aspects of nursing practice.

Because hospitals represent the most structured, concrete, and controlled environment for nursing practice, it is appropriate that associate degree and diploma graduates function well there. Goad (1980) studied the discrepancies between what baccalaureate graduates thought their role in a hospital setting would be and what they actually were required to do in the setting. A recommendation made as an outcome of this study is that "hospitals should explore the use of baccalaureate graduates in roles that differ from associate degree and diploma school graduates" (Goad, 1981, p. 102).

McClure (1978) points out that the 1974 New York State Nurses Association resolution proposing that the baccalaureate degree become the minimal educational preparation for entry into the profession by 1985 was sponsored by the directors of a nursing special-interest group. This leadership group, presumably composed of hospital nursing service administrators to a substantial degree, argues that, because humans are very complex beings, and their needs are made evident in batches that cannot be clearly labeled as "belonging to either the technical or the professional realm," there should be only one level of nurse in the hospital setting—the professional nurse. McClure proposes a model for nursing in which there is no separation of nursing into two dichotomous entities, one professional, one technical; rather, she proposes that professional nursing include technical nursing. McClure (1978, pp. 97–98) reports that the major ideas contained in the proposed revised New York Nurse Practice Act are:

> (1) the requirement of a baccalaureate degree in nursing for all registered nurses *entering* the profession, effective in 1984; (2) the requirement of an associate degree in nursing for all *entering* practical nursing, effective 1984; and (3) transitional mechanisms designed to protect any nurses licensed in either of these two categories prior to the effective date.

Attempts to gain legislative approval of these provisions for changes in the Nurse Practice Act were unsuccessful in 1976, 1978, and 1980.

Thus nursing leaders have differed on the ways in which nurses should be utilized in practice settings. In addition to differing opinions about how nurses should be educated for today's world, there is a continual shift in the health-care needs of society and growing diversity in the roles that nurses hold in the health-care system.

Changes in Nursing's Scope of Practice and Modes of Delivery

An expansion in the roles that nurses can assume has changed the face of nursing markedly. During the late 1960s and through the 1970s, the development of the nurse practitioner roles added even more diversity to nursing's already highly diversified educational system. The typical nurse practitioner role at present includes many elements that are congruent with the professionalization efforts in nursing: greater autonomy and control over one's practice; additional education leading to highly specialized knowledge; opportunity for genuine colleagiality with physicians and other health-care providers; opportunities to practice independently; and increased accountability to clients for the outcomes of nursing care.

Nurse practitioner programs have served as career and educational mobility mechanisms for many registered nurses. With the demise of federal funding, the trend toward placing practitioner programs within existing master's-level programs will undoubtedly accelerate. However, some observers predict that practitioner skills will become more commonly taught in baccalaureate programs (Ford, 1979).

Changing patterns of health-care needs, delivery, and financing are apparent. As our population ages (Metropolitan Life Insurance Company, 1980), meeting the needs of the elderly will become a higher priority. How will these needs be met if Medicaid and Medicare funding diminishes significantly? It appears that national health insurance will not be legislated into existence in the foreseeable future (Prussin, 1978); legislation may encourage increased competition among health-care providers. Will nurses be able to compete successfully for significant portions of the shrinking health-care dollar? What services can nurses provide less expensively, yet with high quality, than any other health-care provider? Many observers believe that nurses are able to provide ambulatory care to well or chronically ill populations at minimum cost with excellent outcomes (Aiken, 1978). Beginning research is being done to test these beliefs (Tomich, 1978, pp. 300–304).

Nurses will continue to be centrally important to the large urban hospitals where major technological advances in health care are in place. Changes in the way traditional nursing care in hospitals is delivered are evident. Probably the most common change is replacing "team nursing" with "primary nursing"—a means of bedside nursing where an individual nurse has round-the-clock responsibility for the planning, implementation, and evaluation of all the nursing care that a patient receives. The primary nurse becomes accountable for the quality of care that the patient receives. This change is consistent with the ANA Standards of Nursing Practice and reportedly results in increased on-the-job satisfaction for hospital nurses, plus better-quality nursing care for patients (Ciske, 1979).

Thus nursing is changing both inside and outside of hospital settings, and those changes seem to be moving inexorably toward greater autonomy for nursing practice, higher standards of education (and thus more education for many nurses), and expanded opportunities for nurses in many different roles in nursing. At no time in our history has it been more important for nurses to reach a consensus on the shape and structure of nursing. If we continue to wrangle with ourselves, it is likely that others will make key decisions for us and at our expense.

Do you believe (as do many people) that "a nurse is a nurse is a nurse?" The lack of differentiation among nurses is an attitude that perhaps stems from our military roots; foot soldiers are interchangeable in the trenches, and maybe nurses are too. This lack of differentiation among nurses with different educational backgrounds pervades nursing service: a nurse with a master's degree in medical surgical nursing may be hired to do the same job, at the same pay, as a nurse with an associate degree. Clearly, they would be able to perform differently, if given the opportunity, but there is an excellent chance that in many hospital settings these two nurses will neither be expected to perform differently, nor allowed to perform differently, nor rewarded for any different performances that they manage to implement.

The roles being taught in an associate degree program and a master's program are *not* the same, however. Educationally mobile nurses have clearly demonstrated this point. If the roles being taught in nursing schools were the same, nurses with an associate degree would very easily complete baccalaureate programs: they would know the nursing role already. As any associate degree graduate who has gone through a baccalaureate program will confirm, the roles taught in the two schools are genuinely different. Certainly there are areas of overlap and duplication, but there are also numerous and critical differences in the nursing roles taught. Both roles are important, valuable, and genuine. That they are *different* does not make one or the other intrinsically better. Nursing will have come of age when differences in roles are congruent in both education and service, when each role is honored for its uniquenesses and contributions to health care, and when each individual who enters nursing can trust that the role being learned has specific career expectations attached to it.

As an educationally mobile nurse, it is important for you to understand the different roles as they exist at this time. It is especially important for you to become an expert in role change. Role change is what returning to school is all about for a nurse. Chapter 4 and all of Part II will more thoroughly explore aspects of role change for educationally mobile nurses.

Impact of Nursing's Evolution on You; You Can Help Change Nursing

This chapter has briefly reviewed some selected aspects of nursing's evolution over the past century. Many evolutionary changes have direct impact upon nurses who are considering or who have actually returned to school. Think about how these changes have had an impact on your life. What is your attitude toward nursing's evolutionary changes? How do you feel about nursing's march toward professionalization? What steps can you as an individual take to help nurses gain consensus about future directions? Do you believe the current status quo is supportable as the way nursing *should* be? What changes would you like to see implemented?

Jot down your answers to these questions now; when you finish your second nursing program, look at these questions and your answers again. Your opinions may or may not change during your school years;

most people's do. Even more important, however, are changes in your commitment to nursing. If your willingness to give time, energy, and money to help nursing move toward a brighter future has increased, then your sojourn in academia will have been successful.

REFERENCES

Aiken, L. "Primary Care: The Challenge for Nursing," in *The Nursing Profession: Views Through the Mist*, ed. N. Chaska. New York: McGraw-Hill Book Co., 1978.

American Nurses Association. *Educational Preparation for Nurse Practitioners and Assistants to Nurses: A Position Paper*. New York: American Nurses Association, 1965.

——. *The American Nurse*, 13, no. 8 (September 1981).

"American Nurses Association's First Position on Education for Nursing," *American Journal of Nursing*, 66 (March 1966), 515–517.

Aydelotte, M. K. "The Future Health Delivery System and the Utilization of Nurses Prepared in Formal Educational Programs," in *The Nursing Profession: Views Through the Mist*, ed. N. Chaska. New York: McGraw-Hill Book Co., 1978.

Brown, E. L. *Nursing as a Profession*. New York: Russell Sage Foundation, 1948.

Bullough, B. "The Associate Degree: Beginning or End?" *Nursing Outlook*, 27, no. 5 (May 1979), 324–328.

Carnegie Commission on Higher Education. *Less Time, More Options*. New York: McGraw-Hill Book Co., 1971.

Ciske, K. L. "Accountability—the Essence of Primary Nursing," *American Journal of Nursing*, 79, no. 5 (May 1979), pp. 891–894.

Conley, V. C. *Curriculum and Instruction in Nursing*. Boston: Little, Brown and Co., 1973.

Etzioni, A., ed. *The Semi-professions and Their Organizations*. New York: The Free Press, 1969.

Ferrell, M. J. *Minimum Behavioral Expectations of New Graduates of New Mexico Schools of Nursing*. Albuquerque, N.M.: University of Albuquerque, 1979.

Flexner, A. *Medical Education in the United States and Canada*. New York: Carnegie Foundation for the Advancement of Teaching, 1910.

Ford, L. C. "A Nurse for All Settings: The Nurse Practitioner," *Nursing Outlook*, 27, no. 8 (August 1979), p. 516.

Gamer, M. "The Ideology of Professionalism," *Nursing Outlook* (February 1979), pp. 108–111.

Ginzberg, E., chairman, Committee on the Function of Nursing. *A Program for the Nursing Profession.* New York: Macmillan, Inc., 1948.

Goad, S. "Role Conceptions Among Baccalaureate Nursing Graduates in Team and Primary Nursing Settings," *Advances in Nursing Science*, 3, no. 3 (April 1981), p. 100.

Jacox, A. "Professional Socialization of Nurses," in *The Nursing Profession: Views Through the Mist*," ed. N. Chaska. New York: McGraw-Hill Book Co., 1978.

Johnson, W. "Advanced Placement in Schools of Nursing: A Statistical Description," in *Open Learning and Career Mobility in Nursing*, ed. C. Lenburg. St. Louis: C. V. Mosby Co., 1975.

———., "Supply and Demand for Registered Nurses. Some Observations on the Current Picture and Prospects to 1985," Part I, *Nursing & Health Care*, 1 (July/August 1980), pp. 16–21.

Kalisch, P. A., and B. J. Kalisch. *The Advance of American Nursing.* Boston: Little, Brown and Co., 1978.

Kohnke, M. F. "Do Nursing Educators Practice What Is Preached?" *American Journal of Nursing*, 73, no. 9 (September 1973), pp. 1571–1575.

Lenburg, C. B. *Open Learning and Career Mobility in Nursing.* St. Louis: C. V. Mosby Co., 1975.

———., and W. Johnson. "Career Mobility through Nursing Education: A Report on NLN's Open Curriculum Project," *Nursing Outlook* (April 1974), pp. 265–269.

McClure, M. "Entry into Professional Practice: The New York Proposal," *The Nursing Profession: Views Through the Mist*, ed. N. Chaska. New York: McGraw-Hill Book Co., 1978.

McQuaid, E. A., and M. T. Kane. "How Do Graduates of Different Types of Programs Perform on State Boards?" *American Journal of Nursing* (February 1979), p. 305.

Merton, R. K. "The Functions of the Professional Association," *American Journal of Nursing*, 58 (January 1958).

Metropolitan Life Insurance Company. *Statistical Bulletin*, 61, no. 1 (January–March 1980), p. 10.

Montag, M. "Looking Back: Associate Degree Education in Perspective," *Nursing Outlook* (April 1980), p. 248.

National Commission on Nursing. *Initial Report and Preliminary Recommendations.* Chicago: Hospital Research and Educational Trust, 1981.

National Joint Practice Commission. *Guidelines for Establishing Joint or Collaborative Practice in Hospitals.* Chicago: The Commission, 1981.

National League for Nursing. *Nursing Data Book: Statistical Information on Nursing Education and Newly Licensed Nurses.* New York: NLN Division of Research, 1978.

Prussin, J. A. "National Health Insurance: A Political Issue at the Crossroads," *Journal of Nursing Administration,* (November 1978), pp. 12–16.

Safier, G. *Contemporary American Leaders in Nursing.* New York: McGraw-Hill Book Co., 1977.

Stein, L. "The Doctor–Nurse Game." *Archives of General Psychiatry,* 16 (1967), pp. 699–703.

Study of Credentialing in Nursing: A New Approach, Volume 1. Report of the Committee. Kansas City, Mo.: American Nurses Association, Publication Code G-1365M, March 1979.

Tomich, J. H. "The Expanded Role of the Nurse: Current Status and Future Prospects," in *The Nursing Profession: Views Through the Mist,* ed. N. Chaska. New York: McGraw-Hill Book Co., 1978.

United States Public Health Service. *Toward Quality in Nursing: Needs and Goals. Report of the Surgeon General's Consultant Group on Nursing.* Washington, D.C.: Government Printing Office, 1963.

Vaughn, J. C. "Educational Preparation for Nursing—1979," *Nursing and Health Care* (September 1980), pp. 80–86.

West, M., and C. Hawkins. *Nursing Schools at the Mid-century.* New York: National Committee for the Improvement of Nursing Services, 1950.

2

Academia: Learning the Lay of the Land

Donna M. Arlton, R.N., M.S., Ed.D.

MOTIVATIONAL FORCES FOR RETURNING TO SCHOOL

In Society

We live in a highly technical, rapidly paced society that places many demands and pressures upon its members. These occur as a result of the rapid changes taking place in many areas of our lives. Some of these changes include an increased expectation for participation in decision making; increased skepticism of the knowledge and skills of experts such as doctors, lawyers, and educators; a growing concern for ecology; a renewed questioning of social values and norms; and a search for personal meaning in life. The list is not complete, but it does attest to the magnitude of the change that surrounds us.

The fast pace of social change challenges the resources of many adults to adapt. This challenge is bringing them back in ever-increasing numbers to continue an education that they thought was completed forever. They are returning to colleges and universities for degrees, extension courses, and adult programs. They undertake both part-time and full-time study; they attend classes on days, evenings, and weekends. They take formal courses, correspondence courses, and telecommunication courses. They represent the fastest growing student population in higher education (Kuntz, 1978).

Many factors motivate adults to return to school. For many middle-aged women who have never worked outside the home, there is a feeling that they lack the identity and tangible rewards associated with a job. Many men also experience a mid-life crisis when they become dissatisfied and seek to escape from what they perceive as dead-end jobs. Young parents, single parents, and empty-nest parents return to school. Minorities are also enrolling in steadily increasing numbers in order to improve their social and economic positions. Continuing education makes it possible for these persons to improve unfavorable life circumstances resulting from a lack of education and preparation.

The knowledge explosion has affected every area of our lives. To be responsible citizens of the communities in which we live, we need to be aware of, and to understand, the many societal trends and issues that affect our daily lives. To effect appropriate social change, we need to understand the workings of our political, educational, and health-care systems. The knowledge explosion has also engulfed the professions. Continuing education has become a necessity for nurses, physicians, lawyers, dentists, engineers, social workers, college professors, and other professionals to practice in a responsible way.

In Nursing

The pressures on nursing to increase its level and quality of education have escalated in recent years. There is much controversy about the state of nursing as a profession. According to Sleicher (1981), nursing has not reached professional status in several areas. It lacks a distinctive body of knowledge; its educational process (the simultaneous existence of hospital-based and collegiate nursing programs) is troublesome; it falls short in the area of autonomy, collegial control, and the provision of a vital social service. Stuart (1981) views professionalism as a scale along which nursing may move. Her concerns are similar to Sleicher's in regard to nursing's need to increase its body of knowledge, the need for greater movement toward collegiate based nursing education, and the need for nursing to become more autonomous. Not until these problems are solved can nursing be truly professional.

At the same time that nursing, as a profession, is being scrutinized and pressured to change, associate degree and diploma nurses may perceive a need to achieve the baccalaureate degree. Many nurses feel threatened by a New York State proposal to increase the minimum preparation for a registered professional nurse to a bachelor of science degree in nursing by 1985. This concept was reaffirmed at the 1978 American Nurses Association convention.

Forces pushing for baccalaureate nursing education come not only from the profession, but from employers as well. Many associate degree and diploma nurses find that positions to which they aspire now require a minimum of a baccalaureate degree. This phenomenon is becoming widespread, especially in supervisory positions, school nursing, and community health settings. A requirement for nurses desiring employment in the Army, Navy, and Air Force is graduation from an NLN-accredited baccalaureate nursing program.

External forces exerted by the profession and employers encourage nurses to return to school. A recent survey of approximately 200 junior-level registered nurse students at Metropolitan State College (1980) in Denver, Colorado, revealed these and other reasons for seeking a baccalaureate nursing degree. Listed in the order most frequently cited, the reasons were as follows:

To obtain a baccalaureate degree because of perceived pressure by the profession.

To become eligible for promotions and supervisory positions.

To prepare for graduate education in nursing practice, education, or administration.

To develop the nursing expertise necessary to function in a community health setting.

To increase nursing knowledge and skill in a current nursing position.

To fulfill a need to learn and to know.

Examination of the reasons cited by associate degree and diploma nurses for returning to school reveals that perceived pressure to obtain a baccalaureate nursing degree ranks first on the list. It is likely that both external pressures and internal needs were operative in the reasons cited for returning to school. In a 1978 article, Kuntz strongly encouraged nurses to return to school. She stated that knowing one's self and enhancing one's knowledge are most worthy goals and will enable the nurse to give better patient care.

SELECTING THE INSTITUTION

If you are a registered nurse seeking a baccalaureate degree, you represent the majority of nurses in the United States today. Almost 80 percent have less than a baccalaureate degree; 11.3 percent have an associate degree and 67 percent have a diploma in nursing (ANA, 1979). Many are returning to school. Many are enrolling in generic programs in nursing. Others are enrolling in B.S.N. programs designed specifically for registered nurse students. Of all the decisions confronting the nurse returning to school, the most critical is the choice of an educational institution. Your state board of nursing may be contacted for a list of accredited programs in your area. If you plan to move to another section of the country, you can obtain, from the National League for Nursing, a list of accredited baccalaureate nursing programs throughout the United States. The material in this section of the chapter will deal with the types of educational institutions and nursing programs available to you.

Four-Year Colleges and Universities

Four-year colleges and universities represent a traditional educational resource. They usually offer on-campus credit programs that are formal, structured, and degree conferring. At the baccalaureate level the major degrees conferred are the bachelor of science and the bachelor of arts degrees. Educational programs of study may vary greatly from one institution to another. Both colleges and universities may be either public or private. Both generally have formal admission requirements that include an evaluation of the high school transcript and transcripts from any other college or university attended. Transfer students may be required to have a C average at the undergraduate level and a B average at the graduate level. In some instances, private institutions are more flexible than public institutions in granting credit for prior education and experience. In addition, the smaller private schools are frequently selected by students desiring a supportive educational environment. Although the cost of tuition at all institutions is rising each year, the tuition at a public college or university is generally much lower than at private schools. However, private schools are often able to offset this difference, particularly to low-income students, by means of a variety of financial aid opportunities.

The manner in which nursing programs are integrated into the university as a whole varies. In large universities, it is customary to find an autonomous College of Nursing, headed by a nurse educator whose title is "dean." In smaller institutions, a Department of Nursing may be one of several units in the School of Health Sciences, the School of Arts and Sciences, the College of Liberal and Applied Arts, or a variety of other arrangements. In these situations, the chief administrative officer of the nursing program may hold the title of "department chairperson," "director," or some other similar title.

Regardless of the structural arrangement of the nursing program within a particular institution, the nursing faculty is accountable for upholding all the policies of the institution. For instance, a particular university may require every graduate to take six credits of history and six credits of mathematics or it may require successful completion of certain tests that indicate competency in specific areas. The nursing faculty cannot ignore these policies, any more than the faculty of the engineering school or the English department can. All-university policies apply to nursing students. It is important for you to know that every nursing program must conform to the policies of the college or university of which it is a part. These constraints cannot be changed unilaterally by the nursing faculty.

Types of Nursing Programs

Whether you choose to attend a college or university, either public or private, you will want to select one that contains a baccalaureate nursing program. You should be aware that there are baccalaureate nursing degree programs and baccalaureate programs for nurses that do not grant nursing degrees. The latter kind of programs frequently grant degrees in areas such as allied health, health-care management, and health education or in behavioral and natural sciences such as psychology, sociology, or biology. These programs frequently appear very attractive to the degree-seeking nurse because they may provide large blocks of blanket credit for prior nursing education, independent study opportunities, off-campus classes, and credit for work experience. In some cases, these programs may be credible. However, the nurse who selects this type of program should understand that the degree conferred is not a baccalaureate nursing degree, and its recipient may be ineligible for entry into a graduate nursing program or for nursing positions in the military service, public schools, community health agencies, and an increasing number of acute-care facilities.

Basically four types of baccalaureate nursing programs were identified by the National League for Nursing open-curriculum study (1977). The first, the licensure-based model, variously known as a "R.N. completion," "upper two," or "second step" program, is designed specifically to meet the educational needs of registered nurse students. In this program, generally characterized by a two-year curriculum, emphasis is placed on treating the R.N. student as an adult learner. There is minimum repetition of previously learned knowledge. Frequently, there is opportunity for R.N. students to attend school on a full-time or part-time basis, and classes may be offered evenings as well as days. The development of this type of program began in the early 1970s and they continue to grow in number.

The second type of nursing program is represented by the advanced placement model. In this nursing program, registered nurses with past education and experience are admitted to advanced standing in generic (basic nursing programs preparing students for licensure) nursing programs. Such academic standing is achieved through transfer credit, credit by examination, or other means such as performance examinations. In some instances, the registered nurse students take classes with the generic students. In others, they have separate classes. This type of program tends to be less flexible than the licensure-based model. It may require more time away from work or a more rigid class schedule, and there is less recognition of previously learned nursing knowledge and skill.

The third type of nursing program allows for multiple exit credentialing and is known as the career ladder model. The career ladder allows for the development of levels of nursing education knowledge and skill, that is, nurse aide, practical nurse, associate, baccalaureate, and master's degree levels. In one model, graduates may exit as nurse aides, practical nurses, or associate degree nurses. In another, they may exit as practical nurses, associate degree, or baccalaureate degree nurses. In a third model, graduates may exit at the associate, baccalaureate, and master's degree levels. There is also a consortium arrangement of career ladder programs wherein a community college offers the associate degree and a four-year college or university offers the baccalaureate and master's degrees. Agreement exists among the consortium institutions as to the program requirements for each of the degree levels. Consortiums exist at the local, state, and regional level.

A fourth type of nursing program selected by practical, associate degree, and diploma nurse-students is the New York Regents External Degree Program. It is unusual because students are awarded a degree upon successful completion of the program's degree requirements, which include demonstration of acquired knowledge through transfer credit or objective assessment procedures. Students who progress through this program tend to be mature, highly motivated nurses who have a strong commitment to nursing and toward continuing professional development. The program, known as an example of the assessment model, makes it possible to earn either an associate or a baccalaureate degree in nursing. The student can choose to meet the program requirements through taking examinations or by doing course work. Most nurses who earn a degree through this program combine courses taken at a college or university with cognitive and performance examinations developed by the nursing faculty and staff of the New York State Regents External Degrees in Nursing Programs. These programs were developed especially to meet the needs of experienced adults who have acquired or wish to acquire college-level knowledge in a variety of flexible ways, including continuing education, work-related experiences, independent study, or college courses (for more information, see Lenburg, 1979, 1980).

Making the initial decision to return to school is a big step. As is true of many adults returning to the academic arena, you may feel overwhelmed with all the decisions to be made and the many changes in your life. You may have many nagging questions, such as "Can I afford to return to school?" "How much time must I study?" "How many courses will I need to take?" "What information must I have if I wish to plan wisely for a return to school?" You will need to establish certain priorities in your life and to set up certain requirements for an acceptable academic program.

In a recent study of 355 registered nurses, Bardossi (1980) found that 57 percent were interested in getting a baccalaureate nursing degree. However, they identified numerous formidable obstacles to the attainment of that goal. The greatest obstacles were time, money, too little credit for past study and experience, and a paucity of convenient programs.

It is not unusual for returning students to make a hurried choice of program based on emotional rather than specific educational factors. Consideration of the following criteria will assist you in the development of a planned selection process that will result in an educationally rewarding back-to-school experience.

Institutions   One of the first decisions you will need to make is whether you wish to attend a university or a four-year college. Do you prefer the advantages of a public or a private institution? Is it important for you to attend an institution with a religious orientation?

Personal mobility is a factor to consider. Are you restricted to a local institution or are you able to move across the country to a desired school? Do you prefer the academic atmosphere of a bustling metropolitan institution or a more tranquil rural academic environment? If you move, what will be the tuition and residency requirements?

Your student colleagues will be an important part of your academic life. Will you be most comfortable in a small school with up to 2,000 students, a medium-sized school with up to 10,000 students, or a large school with over 10,000 students? Does it matter to you what the religious and social makeup of the student body is, what their socioeconomic status and intellectual ability are, and what proportion of them are adult learners?

The educational philosophy of the school you choose may have a strong effect on your self-image as an adult learner. Does it make a difference to you whether the school is very traditional in its approach to teaching and learning or whether it employs a flexible, experimental, adult learner mode of teaching and learning? Do you desire a school where students are encouraged to participate in problem solving and decision making as it relates to curriculum and program matters that affect students?

We live in a time of constantly escalating expenses, and the yearly costs of an academic program are no exception. You will want to examine whether or not the amount of money required for necessary expenses balances the quality of the program. Will it really prepare you for the realities of the profession? Will it open the doors to graduate school? What will you need to pay for books, child care, housing, and food? What share of these expenses must you pay yourself? What financial assistance is available in the form of scholarships, grants, loans, and student work study?

Programs In addition to evaluating the type of institution you desire to attend, you will also want to examine numerous criteria as they relate to the nursing program itself. First, you have the choice of selecting a generic baccalaureate nursing program, one that prepares students for licensure, or you may select a nursing program designed specifically for already licensed associate degree and diploma nurses. The latter type of program frequently provides more flexible learning opportunities for registered nurse students than the former. Clinical resources must be available; be wary of programs that cannot provide you with diverse and rich experiences in community health nursing, as well as sophisticated and up-to-date acute-care experience.

Admission policies, particularly as they relate to application deadlines, transfer of academic credit, entry and challenge examinations, and advanced standing, are important concerns. How many times a year and by what dates are applications for admission accepted? How many and what kind of previously acquired course credits will be accepted by the program? Will you be required to pass cognitive or performance examinations or both prior to being allowed to take nursing courses? If the program is a generic model, can you readily achieve advanced placement in the nursing curriculum through systematic testing or other means, thereby preventing repetition of knowledge and competencies already acquired? How many additional nursing and general education courses will be required for completion of the baccalaureate degree? How many years will be required for you to complete the program? Are there time limits on completing program requirements?

The academic calendar plan and mode of course delivery are other factors to consider. Is the program on a semester, trimester, or quarter system? Are the courses offered each term to facilitate part-time as well as full-time study? Are classes offered evenings and weekends as well as during the day to accommodate the needs of the working registered nurse student?

The reputation of the nursing program will have an impact on your future success in nursing education and practice. You will want to know whether or not the program is accredited by the National League for Nursing. If it is a new nursing program, you will want to determine its potential for being accredited in the near future. You may also have other concerns, such as the following: How do students rate the faculty? What do students say about the curriculum? Do nursing students take the same general education courses as all other students in the institution, or do they take special, perhaps less rigorous, courses planned especially for nurses? Where do its graduates go for further education? What kinds of nursing positions do its graduates obtain? What do employers say about the level of nursing knowledge and skill of the graduates? The school's advising staff should be able to answer these questions; check with experienced students and health-care professionals in the community for their opinions.

The nurse faculty is critical to the success of a nursing program. The following are important questions to consider. Do the terminal degrees of the nursing faculty represent a variety of graduate schools? Does the faculty have advanced education and experience in the areas of their teaching responsibilities? What proportion of the faculty holds doctoral degrees? Do they enjoy the same rights, responsibilities, and privileges as faculty in other areas of the institution? Are faculty members periodically evaluated by students? Is there a sufficient number of faculty to assure well-planned and implemented clinical practicums for students? How much individual attention is provided to students? What kind of grading policies are employed by the faculty?

Last, you will want to evaluate the quantity and quality of counseling services available. Are there enough qualified persons available who can advise you in regard to entry requirements, advanced placement, and allowable credit for prior educational courses? Will the counselor assist you in identifying the complete program of study and in identifying a realistic academic course load?

Student Assistance   When some adult learners return to school, they do not, for a variety of reasons, search for available support services even though they have paid for them with tax dollars and institutional fees. Some of the services that may help you in your role as an adult learner are identified in this section.

Whether you are married or single, with or without children, you may desire to check out the possibility of campus housing. Is it available? Is it less expensive than off-campus housing? Is it spacious enough and comfortable? Is the environment pleasant?

Child care is another service that is essential to many nurse students. You will want to inquire about the hours of operation. What age groups of children will be accommodated? What is the quality of care? How much will it cost?

For many registered nurse-students, returning to the classroom and competing with younger students is frequently very frightening. Because many adult learners have been away from the academic environment for fairly long periods of time, they tend to underestimate their learning abilities and skills. Many can be greatly reassured and benefited through a learning resource center. If you are uneasy about your academic abilities, you might want answers to some of the following questions. Are there either credit or noncredit review and improvement courses available in reading, writing, mathematics, and study skills? Are tutors available? If so, are they knowledgeable about and can they employ adult learning strategies in assisting adult learners to overcome their fears? Are classes available to assist students to reduce test-taking anxieties?

Student health and mental health services should be evaluated. What is the full range of services? How much do the services cost? What is the availability, the benefit, and the cost of student health insurance?

Library resources are an essential part of any academic program. You will want to examine the adequacy of the nursing program holdings. Does the library possess a wide variety of texts, journals, films, filmstrips, transparencies, and other audiovisual media? If not, are those resources available in nearby libraries? Is the library accessible in terms of location and hours of operation? Does it contain comfortable places to study?

Many registered nurse-students require financial aid in one form or another. You will benefit by directing the following inquiries to the financial aid officer of the institution. Am I eligible to receive financial aid? What is the availability of scholarships, grants, loans, work study, and emergency loans? How do I apply for financial aid? What are the advantages and disadvantages of the different types of financial aid?

The use of these criteria will help you to make a well-informed choice about the kind of nursing program you desire to attend. When you are ready to examine a particular nursing program, it is wise to make an appointment with a faculty counselor. You will facilitate the counselor's evaluation of your prior academic program by taking with you all your college or diploma school transcripts. Course descriptions and syllabi are also helpful in making decisions about the kinds and amounts of transfer credit to be allowed.

After you have visited with the faculty counselor, walk around the campus and look at the classrooms, the library, and other points of interest. Talking with students already enrolled in the program is very important and may provide you with insight as to whether or not the program will fit your particular needs.

TYPES OF ACADEMIC CREDIT

The use of the aforementioned criteria for the selection of a baccalaureate nursing program that best meets your needs is vitally important to assure your success in this new and challenging academic venture. However, there is more to consider. Returning nurse-students frequently experience concern and confusion over degree as opposed to continuing education credits, the significance of upper- and lower-division credits, and the difference between quarter and semester credits. In addition, the kinds and amount of academic credits and the strategies for obtaining them may strongly influence the nurse-student in the selection of a nursing program.

Degree versus Continuing Education Credits

To obtain a baccalaureate degree in nursing, you will need to accrue 120 or more semester credits or 180 or more quarter credits. The degree credits in a nursing program are divided between the professional nursing education courses, generally one-third to one-half of the total credits required for the degree, and general education courses. According to the National League for Nursing's "Characteristics of Baccalaureate Education in Nursing" (1979), the first two years of a nursing program consist primarily of courses from the scientific and humanistic disciplines and the last two years of courses in the nursing major. This structure also generally applies to the licensure-based model and the career-ladder type of nursing programs.

Returning nurse-students are sometimes confused about college credit, continuing education participation, and meeting degree requirements. College credits are earned by attending courses that are sponsored or carefully reviewed by an institution of higher learning. Prior to enrolling in a credit-granting course, it should be clearly evident how many college credits are attached to the course. Usually one college credit requires attending class for one hour per week during the sixteen to eighteen weeks of the typical college semester. Classes that contain laboratory experiences may require two to four hours of attendance per week per semester for each credit earned. College credits will be permanently recorded on a student's transcript, kept by the records office of the sponsoring institution.

In contrast, continuing education participation usually does not result in the awarding of college credits. The typical continuing education offering is relatively short and is sponsored by an organization or private group that may have no connection to a college or university. Occasionally, universities and colleges do sponsor continuing education offerings; the announcement of such offerings should clearly spell out whether or not college credit will be awarded. The usual means of documenting attendance at a continuing education offering is the awarding of a certificate, which lists the number of contact hours (these are identical to clock hours) or the number of CEU's (continuing education units). One CEU is equal to ten clock hours.

Because of the differences in control, purpose, length, and type of experience, college credit and continuing education units are not interchangeable. Rarely will a college or university accept continuing education participation as credit toward a degree. It is much more common, however, for college credit to be acceptable for meeting continuing education requirements for relicensure.

When you apply to a college or university for admittance into a degree-granting program, all the transcripts of your college-level work will be reviewed by a program advisor. Each course on your transcript will be reviewed for its equivalency to a course required in the degree-granting program. Only courses that are closely equivalent in terms of general content, scope, requirements, level of difficulty, and quality of instruction will be approved as meeting degree requirements. Some universities have rules regarding how recently the course must have been completed. Courses that are different from the program's requirements, but still acceptable to the university, may be used for meeting *elective* course requirements. Added together, the required courses and the elective courses constitute the total of 120 or more credits needed to graduate from a particular program.

Upper- and Lower-Division Credits

Baccalaureate nursing programs consist of both upper- and lower-division credits. Credits traditionally earned the first two years of a baccalaureate program are called lower-division credits and are characterized by basic courses in general and professional education. Credits earned in the second two years are called upper-division credits and are characterized by more advanced general and professional education content. Courses taken in community colleges provide lower-division credit; associate degrees earned in these institutions are usually composed of only lower-division credit.

It is important for you to recognize that four-year institutions generally place limits on the number of credits, both lower and upper division, accepted for transfer. In addition, there may be certain requirements to be met in the proportion of lower- and upper-division course credits required for the degree. A last point is that you will not be able to substitute lower-division course credits for upper-division credits.

Semester and Quarter Credits

Baccalaureate nursing education programs may operate either on a semester or a quarter system. Programs on a semester system require that students register for classes twice per academic year for two regular semesters of approximately sixteen weeks each. Summer sessions are shorter and may not be required. Programs on a quarter system require registration three or four times per academic year in quarters of approximately ten weeks each.

For some returning students, the conversion of course credits from one system to the other is confusing. The problem will be simplified by the following procedure. To change semester credits to quarter credits, multiply the number of semester credits by one and a half. To change quarter credits to semester credits, multiply the number of quarter credits by 0.66. For example,

$$12 \text{ semester credits} \times 1.5 = 18 \text{ quarter credits}$$
$$18 \text{ quarter credits} \times 0.66 = 12 \text{ semester credits}$$

Grade-Point Averages

Most institutions of higher education assign letter or numerical grades to all students who enroll in a course, indicating the quality of work done by the student. A typical system requires the instructor in a course to devise a grading system that results in an A, B, C, D, or F grade. This is reported to the university registrar, who enters the grade earned on the student's permanent transcript. This letter grade is then transformed to a number, which is then averaged into the other grades the student has earned at that institution. The majority of institutions in this country use a four-point scale for converting letter grades to numbers. In this system, A = 4 points, B = 3 points, C = 2 points, D = 1 point, and F = 0 points. The grade point earned in a particular course is multiplied by the number of credits assigned to the course. For example, if you earned an A grade in a three-credit course, you would receive twelve grade points for your work: $4 \times 3 = 12$. All the grade points earned for a semester are added together and then divided by the total number of credits attempted. The resulting figure is somewhere between 0 and 4.0. The grade-point average you earn at one university is never added to the work you do at a different institution. Each school maintains a running figure that reflects the quality of work you have done at that school only. Furthermore, most institutions do not discount any prior work you have done at their institution. Even if you enrolled in some courses years ago in which you did rather poorly, the grades earned will continue to be reflected in your grade-point average if you return to that same institution.

Transfer and Challenge Credit

You will facilitate your progress through the baccalaureate nursing program by obtaining the greatest possible amount of credit for your prior learning and applying it to the nursing degree requirements. There are two ways this can be accomplished: through the transfer of acceptable credit and by challenge examinations. The remainder of the required credits will have to be earned through enrolling in college courses.

Transfer of credit is the awarding of college credit for equivalent course work taken at another institution of higher education, usually on a course-by-course basis. Transfer credit may be awarded after evaluation of transcripts, catalog course descriptions, and course syllabi. Although some institutions do not place age restrictions on the transfer of college credit, others will not accept credits more than five to ten years old. Transfer credit should not be confused with blanket credit, which is the awarding of college credit for nonequivalent course work, such as the awarding of a single block of credit for a nurse's prior diploma nursing education and work experience. The practice of awarding blanket credit has been prohibited by the National League for Nursing since 1960, because it does not allow for accurate appraisal of the student's nursing knowledge and skill.

You should be aware that academic credit earned in a diploma school of nursing may not transfer to a baccalaureate program, although school policies vary. The reason for the difficulty in transfering credit is that hospitals are accredited to provide health-care services, but not academic degrees. Hospitals are not eligible to join consortia through which institutions of higher education develop policies and agreements about how credits will transfer. Generally, colleges and universities will accept as transfer credit only those credits earned in other colleges or universities. Diploma nurses frequently may obtain college credit through challenge exams.

The challenge examination is a vehicle whereby students gain academic credit by taking an examination on the content of a course offered by the school. If the student passes the exam, academic credit is awarded. Challenge exams may be given for both general education and nursing courses; they may be made by the local teachers at an institution or they may be developed by committees composed of educators from around the country; they may be required by a particular school either before or after admission. Teacher-made exams usually have been reviewed only by the students in the school, and the questions reflect the content taught in that particular course. The tests constructed by national committees include those provided through the American College Testing Program (ACT), which uses tests developed by the New York State Education Department and the Regents External Degree Programs, College Level Examination Program (CLEP), and the National League for Nursing (NLN). These tests are known as "standardized" tests, because they have been carefully constructed to reflect widely accepted facts and procedures, and they have been given to large numbers of students in different regions of the country. The scoring of such tests is based upon how large numbers of students performed on the test.

Most challenge examinations assess knowledge; however, some nursing programs also assess clinical performance skills through teacher-prepared written simulations, simulated clinical laboratories, and direct observation of students in the clinical setting. The Regents External Degrees in Nursing Program at the University of the State of New York has developed objective, criterion-referenced nursing performance examinations. These examinations represent an attempt to make performance testing as reliable, fair, and thorough as written tests. Some nursing programs require students to pass clinical performance and/or written challenge examinations to "validate" their prior nursing education, as well as to provide credit toward a degree.

Before you make a final commitment to any nursing program, become knowledgeable about the institution's policies regarding the kinds and amounts of transfer and challenge examination credit you can be awarded toward the nursing degree. Ask the advisor for the nursing program or scour the written documents the program provides to prospective students. Careful attention to the other criteria listed in this chapter will help you to select the nursing program best suited to your personal and nursing education needs. Good luck to you in your great adventure!

REFERENCES

American Nurses Association. "National Sample Survey of Registered Nurses," *American Nurse*, 11, no. 1 (May 1979).

Bardossi, K. "Why BSN Programs Drive Nurses Crazy," in *A Comprehensive Guide to Part-Time BSN Programs: A Presentation of RN Magazine*. Reprinted from *RN Magazine* (February–March 1980), pp. 3–5.

Kuntz, B. "Returning to School," *Supervisor Nurse* (February 1978), pp. 15–17.

Lenburg, C., ed. *Open Learning and Career Mobility in Nursing.* St. Louis: C. V. Mosby Co., 1975.

——."Emphasis on Evaluating Outcomes: The New York Regents External Degree Program," *Peabody Journal of Education* (April 1979), pp. 212–221.

——."In Search of the BSN: How to Decide Which Program Does You Justice," *RN* (February–March 1980), pp. 10–13.

Metropolitan State College. "Registered Nurse Student Survey." Unpublished, Denver, Colo., 1980.

National League for Nursing. *Characteristics of Baccalaureate Education in Nursing*, Pub. No. 15-1758. New York: The League, 1979.

Sleicher, M. A. "Nursing Is Not a Profession," *Nursing and Health Care*, 2, no. 4 (April 1981), pp. 186–191.

Stuart, G. W. "How Professionalized Is Nursing?" *Image*, 13, no. 1 (February 1981), pp. 18–23.

3

Searching for Financial and Workplace Resources

Karen Bergman Tomajan, R.N., B.S.N.
Martha Albert, Ph.D.
Donea L. Shane, R.N., M.S.

This chapter will briefly discu   some conventional and unconventional sources of support for the edu   tionally mobile nurse.

STUDENT FINANCIAL AID

Your first stop in your search for financial support should be the financial aid office at the school you have chosen to attend. In the past, federal nurse training acts have generously supported nurses who wanted to further their education. Unfortunately, those golden days have passed, and finding federal- or state-supported educational grants or loans will be much more difficult (if possible at all).

The application mechanism for federally supported loans is quite lengthy, so be sure to ask about deadline dates. You will be required to divulge your full financial situation as a part of the application process. Most federal support for education is earmarked for beginning students from low-income families; thus it may be impossible for you to qualify for many of the assistance programs.

Your school may have a scholarship fund for deserving students. Ask at the financial aid office about such funds and what the criteria for award are. Again, there may be a long waiting period between the deadline for application and the announcement of awards.

Some nursing schools have separate scholarship funds that are privately donated. Check with the nursing school you will be attending to learn about the application process for these awards.

Special Scholarships

You may be eligible for some specialized assistance that you are not aware of presently. Specialized scholarship programs are usually connected with social clubs, union membership, veterans organizations, religious groups, or an ethnic origin group. Since some of these scholarship programs are not well publicized, you will need to do some research to find out about them. Visit a college library to check out one of the several books that list current scholarships. It is also possible to have a search done for you by a private firm, for a fee ranging from $40 to $50 in most cases. Such firms usually advertise in the yellow pages of metropolitan telephone directories, in weekly newspapers connected with colleges, and sometimes in magazines aimed at the typical college-age student or their parents. *Caution*: Avoid firms that charge very high fees, sometimes up to $1500.

Professional nursing organizations also sponsor scholarships. The American Nurses Foundation, which is closely allied with the American Nurses Association, has an active scholarship program for which you may be eligible. Several nursing specialty organizations also sponsor scholarships for members who are furthering their education. Information on these programs is usually available through the publications sponsored by the associations. Local hospital or medical society auxiliaries may sponsor scholarships. Inquire through their officers.

Loans

Loans may be available to you, at slightly lower interest rates than loans for new cars, through state or federal tax-supported programs. Your state or district nurses association may sponsor a loan fund for members. Clearly understand when you must start repaying the loan. Interrupting your enrollment may make it immediately payable. Read the fine print in any contract you sign. Know exactly how much the interest rate is, how much the monthly pay-back payment will be, and whether there are penalties for rapid repayment. Private banks may loan money for education, also. The interest rate on this money may be slightly higher than for loans subsidized by state or federal government money. If you must borrow money to finance your education, *comparison shop*. Interest rates may vary significantly. Some loans can be forgiven if you work in a certain area or at a certain institution for a period of time.

Be wary of borrowing money from more than one source. When you graduate, each source will expect you to start paying back the loans immediately, so your monthly payment can be quite large. It may be cheaper and more realistic for you to borrow the full amount from one source and pay it back over a longer period of time than to make several small loans that must all be paid back in a short amount of time.

Family Financial Resources

Unquestionably, the present era is characterized by diminishing sources of free education for students. More than at any time in the past quarter-century, students and their families will have to assume the full responsibility for paying for higher education. Here are some pertinent questions for you and your family to consider:

Do we have any assets that can be sold? Jewelry, inherited property, a rental house, collections, or art?

Do we have an inheritance to borrow against or parents willing to extend money in advance?

Can we take out a second mortgage on our house? If we do borrow money in this fashion now, will anticipated higher incomes later compensate for current interest rates on borrowed money?

Can we "income average" on our federal income tax? In certain tax brackets, this acts like a federal tax subsidy for a family.

To make knowledgeable decisions about these complex financial matters, you would be wise to consult an accountant familiar with your family's total financial situation.

To Work or Not to Work

This indeed is a knotty question. Perhaps you have no choice in the matter; you must work a certain amount to keep your family financially afloat. If you have some leeway financially, you would probably be wise to reduce your workplace commitments to the minimum amount you can afford during your return-to-school days. You will progress faster through school and thus be able to return to work more quickly on a full-time basis. Furthermore, your stress level may be significantly less. Remember, however, that your loss of income is a real cost; it may be the major cost of returning to school. You should assume that your enhanced educational credentials will provide opportunities for higher paying jobs. Thus your cost–benefit analysis must weigh the probability of higher income later against the short-term reduced income while you are in school. Your payoff, in terms of learning and professional outcomes, are also benefits you reap by returning to school. They are hard to assign dollar values to, however.

Many nurses work full time while taking one or two prerequisite courses per semester. This is a very reasonable plan if you cannot cut back on your employment responsibilities at present. This lengthens the total amount of time you spend getting your new degree, of course, but it is a reasonable way for easing into the student role. In some programs it is necessary to spend one or two semesters in full-time study. If you simply cannot afford to cut back on your full-time job, you will need to be very creative in how you manage those two full-time commitments. First, you might save up vacation days, then take them off one per week (assuming you are on a typical five day per week schedule.) Second, investigate how you can get around the school's full-time semester plan. This may mean taking only half a level (or course, or year) per calendar year. But if it is the *only* way for you to accomplish your goal, try it! Those years you spend going very slowly toward your goal are more productive in the long run than complaining about not being able to go, and thus getting nowhere.

Employee Tuition Reimbursement Plans

Where you work may be as important a question as *whether* you will work while in school. The right employment situation while you are in school can be an invaluable resource in helping you meet your educational goals. Fortunately, as the nursing shortage becomes more critical, hospitals are recognizing that to help nurses meet their educational goals can be an important device for recruitment and retention. In fact, a survey done by the National Association of Nurse Recruiters (1981) notes that the number one recruitment tool and the number two retention tool is tuition reimbursement. Furthermore, hospitals are recognizing that supporting educational mobility is a good way to develop future managers from among their present nursing staff members. This modeling effort within an institution can inspire others to advance.

Our advice is to work for an institution that will actively help you to meet your educational goals. In terms of tuition reimbursement, find the answers to these questions:

What percentage of your school tuition will the employer pay?

What limits are there on the amount of tuition reimbursement per year?

How long must you work for the employer before you are eligible for tuition reimbursement?

Will you owe the employer a certain amount of time as an employee as a payback mechanism? If you must leave the employer before this obligation is fulfilled, what monetary costs will you incur? Will there be a penalty or higher than usual interest rate tacked on to the principal?

When does the tuition reimbursement occur? Is it *after* you have received a grade in the course? Obviously, in this case, you will have to come up with the tuition money yourself at registration time. Your employer will be reimbursing you after you finish a semester.

Is your choice of school limited under the employer's reimbursement plan?

Will the fees for challenge examinations be reimbursed?

Must you be continuously enrolled under the reimbursement plan, or can you take a semester or two off without having to reapply or begin repayment of your obligation?

Is there a limit to the amount of college credits your employer will allow you to take per semester or year?

Where is the tuition reimbursement money coming from? Is there a limited pool of money that might dry up before you have reached your goals? Is there a competitive mechanism for deciding which employees will receive limited tuition reimbursement funds?

Tuition reimbursement plans may differ markedly, even among the institutions in a single community. Investigate carefully.

OTHER WAYS YOUR EMPLOYER CAN HELP

Financial support is not the only way your employer can help you to achieve your educational goals. As an exemplar of what employers can do to help nurses meet their educational mobility goals, we will share with you the Educational Mobility Program developed by the Department of Nursing Career Development at Presbyterian Hospital in Oklahoma City, Oklahoma. The key element in this program is the educational mobility counselor employed by the hospital. This person works with potential and long-term employees, schools in the area, and the local nursing professional associations in order to provide meaningful information, strong support systems, role models, and communication networks for educationally mobile employees.

The educational mobility counselor assists nurse–employees in making contact with college representatives in the immediate area. This may include planning periodic "education days" when school representatives come to the hospital to speak individually with interested nurses. Alumni and current students are included in the program as valuable resource people.

Because of the educational mobility counselor's experience and familiarity with area schools, concrete help can be given in goal clarification (for those nurses who have not yet committed themselves to returning to school), course planning, and work scheduling. The realities of time management are explored with each individual. How many hours can be worked per week during a semester in which the nurse-student is enrolled in six college credits of course work? This varies, of course, from person to person, but experience strongly suggests that six credits is the upper limit for a full-time worker. This may be too many for individuals who have unusual home stresses, moderate academic skills, or an especially demanding position within the hospital.

The educational mobility counselor can introduce an employee to the communication-and-support network that has been developed and meets regularly at the hospital. This support group can help employees make the tension-filled adjustment to the student role. Specific help can be given during times that are predictably stressful. One peak stress time is when an individual is completing entrance exams, which may include clinical performance tests. Group help at this time reassures an individual that *everyone* becomes very anxious during critical evaluations. A library of current nursing references is helpful. Sharing materials on or accounts of the process can be supportive. Tutoring, perhaps in writing nursing care plans, can be provided. Nurse specialists employed in the institution could give review and update sessions in their specialty.

On occasion, the educational mobility counselor is able to arrange for in-hospital offerings of required courses. In those schools in which independent study courses are available, groups can be organized to proceed through these courses together.

Flexible staffing is a critically important opportunity that can be offered by employers to educationally mobile nurse employees. Such staffing patterns may be the single most important ingredient in a nurse's decision to return to school. Flexible staffing may include lengthening the average work day from eight to ten or twelve hours, thus reducing the number of days per week one must work. It may mean changing some staffing rules about how days off are allocated, thus allowing nurse–students the same days off each week during the semester. It may mean introducing special weekends-only schedules for full-time pay. Flexible staffing and a willingness to recognize the scheduling difficulties students may experience can serve as strong support systems to the educationally mobile employed nurse.

Impact of Employers' Involvement in Educational Mobility

Hospitals and other health-care employers are realizing that the recruitment of nurses to their staffs can be enhanced by helping employees meet their educational goals. Because educationally mobile nurses are motivated individuals who are typically interested in advancing patient care and professional nursing, the recruitment of these extra-special nurses is obviously to the advantage of an employer. Furthermore, an active educational mobility program within an employing institution can help retain nurses who might otherwise move to a hospital that does offer better tuition reimbursement, educational support, or communication networks.

Probably the most important outcome of an educational mobility program is an improvement in patient care. Nurses in such programs will be more likely to apply concepts being learned in school. They will usually have clinical experiences in other hospitals and institutions and will have worked with other nurses (either as fellow students or while in clinical experiences); thus they are exposed to new ideas about health care that are being implemented in the local community. Their class work—papers, research projects, care plans—can be directly applied to patient care.

Another potentially important outcome of employers' involvement in educational mobility programs is that the gap between nursing service and nursing education can be lessened. By working cooperatively on a program, the educators and administrative nurses will come to a clearer understanding of the needs and values of each group.

Finally, by nurturing the development of presently employed staff members, an institution's leadership group can be advanced from within the organization. This has benefits in terms of the knowledge of the setting this permits. It also saves the expense of hiring outside consultants or specialists for leadership searches, and it may significantly improve the morale within an organization.

An Advocate for the Educationally Mobile Employee

At Presbyterian Hospital in Oklahoma City, the educational mobility counselor maintains an open dialogue with nursing schools and becomes familiar with requirements, curricula, and key personnel. The educational mobility counselor serves on planning committees in the local nursing schools, providing input from the standpoint of the employed educationally mobile nurse. Assistance is given to any staff member considering a return to school, and continuous contact is maintained with students once they have made the decision to enroll and are progressing through the steps necessary to earn the degree. Membership in career ladder organizations and professional societies is maintained in order to keep abreast of trends in the profession that affect educational mobility.

All this adds up to providing an advocate for the educationally mobile nurse employee. We suggest that you search for an employer who can provide this kind of support for you.

If none is available, perhaps you can be influential in developing an advocacy role in your present environment. Try stimulating interest in the development of a support network in your favorite workplace. Discuss ideas with nursing leaders, such as supervisors, the director of nursing, or the in-service educators your institution employs. Since nearly every hospital in the country is affected by the nursing shortage, employers may welcome ideas that offer realistic ways for improving their recruitment and retention rates.

Second, you might investigate moving to a location in which a supportive employing institution is available. Your long-term career development may make such a move very worthwhile. Men in our society have always had the privilege of moving to an advantageous job location. Perhaps the time has arrived when female nurses should have this opportunity.

Third, you might approach your local professional association. Your nurse colleagues who have joined together in the association may be able to help organize the needed support networks in employing institutions. The professional associations may have advisory councils, joint committees, or other organizational mechanisms for cooperative interface between schools and employers.

SUMMARY

If the will is strong enough, almost always a way can be found to acquire an academic degree in nursing. The attainment of additional education is a priceless possession in many ways. Remember this as you take Aunt Hattie's wedding present Ming vase to the auction block. Education *will* be worth the sacrifice.

REFERENCES

National Association of Nurse Recruiters. *Recruitment Survey, June 1981*. Provided by *Nursing 81*.

4

Role: A Look at Role Theory and Role Change

Judith Maurin, R.N., Ph.D.

This chapter will provide an overview of role theory: what roles are, how they are acquired and changed, and the impact of these processes upon the individual. Therefore, this discussion can be generalized to situations other than returning to school. Some individuals may find such abstractness frustrating. You may ask, "Why bother with role theory?" There are two reasons. First, we know quite a bit about how roles are acquired and changed. An understanding of these processes will help you understand what you are experiencing as you return to school. By putting your experience into a broader framework, you may be able to gain more objectivity about a very personal experience. Being able to make sense out of an experience is a big first step in coping with it. Second, your understanding of these processes could help you to help others. Many people that nurses deal with are struggling with role change too. If you can generalize the core characteristics of the concept of role change to specific examples, you will have gained a theoretical perspective for understanding what many of your clients are experiencing.

As you progress through your student experiences, some stress and conflict is to be expected. Much of this is the result of your changing roles. Some students will experience more stress than others, because the nature and extent of change required when returning to school varies with the individual. Others around you will also experience stress and strain, because the changes you make in your life require them to change theirs.

This is not the first time you have experienced role change, nor will it be the last. When you complete the program and return to the world of work, you will be a changed person; again, the old working relationships will have to be revised. An understanding of role relationships will therefore be useful to you now and throughout the rest of your life.

ROLE: A BRIDGING CONCEPT

Role is a useful concept because it is a bridging concept. It provides a bridge between society and the individual. We participate in society through the enactment of roles, since social structures are made up of roles and role relationships. Something as abstract as an organization's hierarchical structure comes alive through the activity of many individuals enacting their roles and participating in interdependent role relationships. This participation, in turn, contributes to the formation of our "self," who we come to see ourselves as and the value we assign ourselves.

There are different theoretical perspectives from which to study role, and each emphasizes a selected focus. See Hardy and Conway (1978, Chapter 2) for a discussion and differentiation of two important perspectives for the study of role, the *functionalist* and the *symbolic interactionist* perspectives. This discussion will draw from both, first presenting role as an aspect of society and then discussing the implications for self.

SOCIAL ROLES

From the point of view of society, *roles* are more or less fixed positions to which certain expectations and demands are attached. (Think of role in the abstract, minus any particular person who fills it.) The expected behaviors of a role are defined by *norms*, rules that prescribe and/or proscribe how one should act, think, and feel while assuming that role. For example, some of the common norms associated with the role of nurse include these: a nurse should perform the self-care activities that the client is unable to perform, no matter how intimate the activity; a nurse should bring scientific knowledge to bear on assessment data, in order to recognize problems and formulate goals for the client; a nurse should not feel sexually attracted to a client. You may resist the idea that there are norms about how one should feel while enacting a role. However, it is precisely because we have learned such norms that we feel so guilty when we encounter proscribed feelings in ourselves. Why else would we have to work so hard just to identify negative feelings in ourselves before we can deal with them? Why else would we call them "negative" feelings? Although some norms are learned through direct instruction, most are acquired outside of our awareness through *socializing agents* that apply negative and positive sanctions to produce the expected (desired) behavior from us in a role. Negative sanctions are conditions that punish or discourage performance, and positive sanctions are conditions that reward or encourage performance.

Who are socializing agents? Any role partner is a socializing agent, because all of these people are giving subtle (and sometimes not so subtle) messages about whether your behavior is meeting their expectations. Obviously, your teachers are giving you messages about how well you are performing as a student, but so are your classmates. If you do not pull your weight on a group project, or if your class participation always gives evidence that you have done extra reading, you are very likely to hear about it from classmates. In this way your classmates, too, socialize you to what is acceptable "student behavior" in this group.

Why should socializing agents be so abundant? It is important to your role partners that you perform your role as they expect, because roles are reciprocal. *Reciprocity* means that role partners are mutually dependent upon one another for the successful performance of their roles. They cannot perform their role as they want to if you do not perform yours in the way they expect. For example, if a good mother is one who can satisfy the needs of her infant, a new mother cannot feel like a "good mother" if her baby is colicky or unresponsive. In this situation, the baby is not being the expected role partner. The baby is not performing the expected or desired behaviors that let mother know that she is a good mother. Likewise, a person cannot be "teacher" if the role partners refuse to be "students."

When we add the concept of *role set*, you can see the complications of this characteristic of reciprocity. A role set is the constellation of relationships with the role partners of a particular position. As student, for example, you usually engage in role relationships with multiple others (teachers, classmates, secretaries, librarians, and so on). Because of reciprocity, all these role partners are dependent upon you performing your role in a way which will complement theirs. When these multiple role partners conflict over the role performance they expect from you, social interaction may be stressful indeed.

To complicate matters even further, no individual occupies just one role. A woman may be a wife, mother, nurse, artist, and so on. Because you occupy a cluster of roles, you also have a cluster of role partners and expectations for your behavior that are likely to conflict at times. For example, have you experienced times when your role partners at home expected you to be "wife" or "husband," "mother" or "father," when you felt the need to be "student"? Try to identify the negative sanctions you received—a hurt look, a cutting remark. Likewise, you have probably received positive sanctions as well—the provision of quiet study time, or hearing your spouse brag to a friend that you are at the university working on a degree.

Up to this point, we have been concentrating on role expectations: what society tries to get from the individual. However, role performance (what society actually gets) depends upon many factors. An important factor is the meaning we attribute to the situation we are in and to the messages we receive. As human beings, we do not only respond to stimuli; we select and interpret stimuli as well. We do not just react, we initiate behavior as well. Meanings and values are part of a group's culture and are learned from the individuals with whom we interact (Stryker, 1959, p. 114).

> Humans respond to a classified world, one whose salient features are named and placed into categories indicating their significance for behavior. In short, humans do not respond to the environment as physically given, but to an environment as it is mediated through symbols—to a *symbolic environment.* Persons frequently enter situations in which their behavior is problematic. Before they can act, they must define the situation, that is, represent it to themselves in symbolic terms. The products of this defining behavior are termed "definitions of the situation."

Social interaction proceeds through the use of symbols that have meaning for individuals and call forth a response based on those meanings. Each actor takes the other into account by interpreting (imputing meaning to) the symbols and actions used by the other during the course of interaction. Communication and sustained interaction are possible when individuals possess a system of shared meanings. The absence of a system of shared meanings results in confusion, misunderstanding, and the inability to sustain interaction. This often occurs between persons of different cultural or subcultural groups.

Our position in the social structure and the resulting consequence an event has for us because of this position also contribute to the definition of a situation. As American middle-class parents, for example, we have probably learned to value curiosity and an inquiring mind in a child. Imagine such a three-year-old female child. She asks numerous questions and enjoys manipulating objects to see what will happen. Accompanying this child are two adult women, one the child's mother and the other, a visiting friend. If asked whether they value intellectual curiosity in a child, each woman is likely to answer "yes." Yet each may very well define this child's behavior differently, because of their differing social positions. One would not be surprised if the mother defined the child's behavior as exasperating and harmful, since in her position she must assume the responsibility for protecting the child and household belongings from the child's curiosity. The visiting friend, free of responsibility for the child, may also be more free to enjoy and appreciate this "bright little girl." Each woman is observing the very same behaviors, but because of the different meanings these behaviors have for each woman, their behaviors toward the child will be different.

The likelihood of situations being defined differently, depending upon one's social position, can lead to strained interactions and wrongful imputing of motives to role partners. A good example is the challenge exam, which is frequently used by schools to assess prior knowledge. The faculty perceives expectations (from colleagues in their school, in the wider university, and from accrediting bodies) that certain standards be enforced. They also perceive expectations from applicants that learning experiences not be repetitive. Since nurses returning to school come with such different levels of ability and prior experience, the challenge exam looks like a logical solution. The faculty sees these exams as a way to demonstrate that it adheres to high standards, while allowing for student differences. The educationally mobile nurses come to this situation knowing their abilities and past experiences, and with the usual anxieties most of us experience in a testing situation. They are acutely aware that the balance of power in this relationship is with the faculty—a vulnerable feeling.

From this position, it is easy for the students to impute motives to the faculty which say that the faculty devises challenge exams because it does not value the experience of the nurse and assumes the nurse is ignorant until proved otherwise. The faculty encounters the resulting hostility with surprise (after all, they have put a great deal of effort into developing and providing this opportunity to meet requirements quickly) and imputes motives to the students such as "wanting everything easy" and "wanting to hide what they do not know." And so the interaction deteriorates with the possibility of achieving a "self-fulfilling prophecy" by creating the attitudes and behaviors in the other that were wrongfully imputed at the start. When role partners are in differential positions of power vis-à-vis one another, the situation is ripe for widely different meanings being attributed to the situations in which these role partners find themselves interacting.

The teacher–student role is by no means unique in that the role partners possess unequal shares of the power. As nurses we routinely participate in many such relationships, sometimes on one side of the power balance and sometimes on the other. For example, the nurse who is caring for a patient having "minor" surgery may learn that the patient does not define the need for any surgery as minor. Once again, role partners in differential positions of power have failed to agree on the meaning of the situation.

When it comes to role performance, society does not get conformity from us in all our roles. In fact, a process of role negotiation is going on between us and our role partners. This negotiation is accomplished through the processes of *role taking* and *role making*.

"Role-taking refers to anticipating the responses of others implicated with one in some social act" (Stryker, 1959, p. 115). This is an empathic ability that enables you to imagine yourself in the place of the other or to imagine how the other understands your communication. Role taking enables you to anticipate the response of your role partner to your behavior, thereby facilitating role performance. For example, as a nurse doing health teaching with a client, you imagine the world of experience of your client, selecting examples and language accordingly. You further imagine how those examples were understood; this image then guides subsequent health teaching behavior. The ability to accurately engage in role taking is partially a learned skill and partly a function of what is going on with you in the specific interaction. Anxiety may produce a perceptual distortion, which interferes with an individual's role-taking ability.

We do not always enact roles as we imagine the role partner expects, however. We may negotiate roles through the process of role making. Role expectations are seldom so fixed that there is no room for individual interpretation. Role making also involves anticipating the response of the other, but one structures the interaction so as to modify the expected role in some way (Turner, 1962, pp. 20–40). When the behavior of a role partner departs from the one anticipated in some segment of the interaction, the other may apply a negative sanction and even terminate interaction; or the other may accept the change so that interaction is sustained. In the latter case, role making can be said to have taken place.

ROLES AND IDENTITY

You will remember that role is a bridging concept. It is by means of roles that we participate in society, and our participation in these roles in turn contributes to the formation of one's self. Take a moment now to write twenty answers to the question, "Who am I?"

Were you able to come up with twenty? More? Research has shown that people are more likely to respond with a list of nouns than adjectives, and these nouns are usually roles that are very important to them (husband, wife, architect, nurse, and so on). Therefore, the roles we play are important, because they become integrated into our identity (Kuhn and McPartland, 1967, p. 120). Mead expresses this idea in his discussion of the self as composed of the "me" and the "I." The "me" corresponds to the sum of the roles one defines as one's own. We have a defined "me" for each of our roles. "An individual's various 'me's' are seen by him, not only as discrete objects; he may perceive all of them at once and in a hierarchy, according to the degree of positive attitude he holds toward them" (Rose, 1980, p. 44). The "me" is the organized attitudes and expectations of others that the individual himself assumes. The "I" is the personal, unique aspect of the self. It is one's perception of oneself as a whole, as more than the role one plays. It is the individual's response to the attitudes of the others.

> In sum, the individual has parts of himself which are reflections of his relationships with others, and which others can take the role of and predict fairly accurately how the individual is going to behave in the relationship. There is another part of the individual—his self-conception—the attitudes of which may be, in part, assigned by the individual to himself, and which are not necessarily expected in the culture. This personal self-conception may be conformist as well as deviant, and while it is always subject to change, it is often stable enough for another person to predict fairly accurately what behavior the individual will engage in, even aside from the cultural expectations for his roles. The "I," while personal, is by no means independent of cultural expectations, since it is built on the individual's "me's," and since the individual always sees himself in relation to the community.

There are both content and evaluative aspects to our identity (the roles we play). We give a value to ourselves and our roles, just as we evaluate other objects. This, too, is in part a consequence of social interaction and the process of reflexive role taking. In reflexive role taking, we use our role partner as a mirror, reflecting the expectations and/or evaluations of the self as seen by the other (Cooley's "looking-glass self," 1902).

In reflexive role taking, the individual is focused upon how he appears to the other, and shapes his behavior in an attempt to elicit an evaluation from the other that is consistent with the evaluation he has learned to value. For example, the new nurse on a unit will note the words, expressions, and behaviors of the head nurse, fellow staff nurses, physicians, and patients for clues about how they are evaluating the new employee. It would be hard to think of yourself as a competent staff nurse or to feel good about yourself if you kept perceiving negative evaluations from your important audiences. A general principle found in the literature on socialization is that "other things being equal, the greater the consistency, duration, and intensity with which a definition is promoted by others about an actor, the greater the likelihood that an actor will embrace that definition as truly applicable to himself" (Lofland, 1969, p. 121).

Interactions vary in the extent to which the evaluation and definition of self is an issue. Turner (1970) identified two types of interpersonal interactions: *task oriented* and *identity oriented*. Task-oriented interactions are directed toward a goal. Role taking is required to imagine how the other person understands your communication and acts so that collaboration can occur and the goal be achieved. Identity-oriented interactions are primarily influenced by one or both partner's concern about how one partner feels toward the other, with the attitude sought being that which supports one's self-conception. The role taking here is imagining what meanings and values the other is attributing to one's self. Preoccupation with self in the identity-oriented interaction means that an individual is attending to the other's gestures primarily for a clue as to how the other views him. Any task, if there is one in this interaction, becomes secondary.

At times an interaction may start out task oriented, but become identity oriented. Three conditions that may trigger such a shift are the following:

1. If one or both actors enter the interaction very insecure and self-conscious.
2. If one or both actors have learned from past experience to be on guard for attack (devaluation or refusal to validate one's self-conception) from the other.
3. If difficulty with task completion leads the participants to look for explanations for the failure in the personal characteristics of the other (assigning blame).

Finally, not all roles and the expectations associated with them are voluntarily accepted. Some roles may be seen as alienating, because they are imposed upon their incumbents; there is an attempt to coerce identification with roles or groups one does not wish to join (Holland, 1977). For some, returning to the student role may have an aspect of this quality. Whether an instructor's lecture assumes you are all beginning students with no nursing experience, or whether upon leaving your biology class you hear another student say, "If you are a woman in this class, it is hard to be taken seriously, because it is assumed you are just a nursing student," the label you feel yourself being given can be very hard on your identity.

This identity aspect of role taking is very important in the genesis of the self during childhood socialization and in adulthood when encountering new situations in which we are unsure of ourselves. Think about your experiences connected with returning to school. You ought to be able to identify at least a few experiences (perhaps when you were interacting with a teacher, a beginning nursing student, or another experienced nurse) when you were very sensitive to the impression you were making, and you were watching that other person for a reaction to you. That was an identity-oriented interaction.

ROLE CHANGE

Role change consists of adding a new role, dropping an old role, or modifying the behaviors associated with a role already a part of a role cluster. Objectively, the process of role change is no different than the processes we have already discussed. What usually makes role change problematic is, first, the phenomenon of reciprocity, which means that the impact of our behavior change ripples through all our role partners, and, second, the resulting identity adjustment that goes with it. Imagine that a staff nurse decides to modify the staff nurse role by incorporating assertive, professional judgments about what is quality patient care. Instead of nodding when the physician says a patient is not to be told his diagnosis, this nurse shares the assessment that, while he will undoubtedly need support, his repeated requests for information indicate a readiness to confront the truth. Or when the intern prescribes two drugs known to interact negatively, this nurse points out the error, instead of "forgetting to give it" until the intern's supervisor can discover the mistake. Imagine the impact such a modification would have for the the nurse's various role partners. This staff nurse may well encounter outrage toward the new behavior before realizing new respect. You can also imagine that this nurse's self-image could change as a result.

ROLE STRESS
AND ROLE STRAIN

The problems one encounters in participating in roles can best be discussed through the concepts of role stress and role strain. "Role stress is a social structural condition in which role obligations are vague, irritating, difficult, conflicting, or impossible to meet" (Hardy and Conway, 1978, p. 76). Role stress refers to the characteristics of a situation in which resource excesses or deficits of the role occupant(s) and/or characteristics of the system make role demands difficult or impossible to meet. The types of role stress that have been identified include role ambiguity, role incongruity, role conflict, role overload, role incompetence, and role overqualification. The definitions of these situations of role stress come from Hardy and Conway (1978, pp. 81–88).

Role ambiguity   role expectations are vague, ill defined, or unclear, and therefore sanctions may be inconsistent and haphazardly applied.

Role conflict   role expectations are contradictory or mutually exclusive.

Role incongruity   role expectations demand behavior that runs counter to the role occupant's self-perception, disposition, attitudes, and/or values.

Role overload   role demands are excessive so that, whereas a role occupant could competently perform each role demand, the occupant is unable to perform them all in the time available.

Role incompetence   the role occupant's resources are inadequate relative to the demands of the role.

Role overqualification   the role occupant's resources are in excess of those required for the role.

As Hardy and Conway (1978) point out, in any specific example of role stress, it is often difficult to sort out the part that the social structure plays in creating role stress from that played by the individual's resource level. For example, role overload could occur when two job positions are needed in place of the excessive demands for one, or it could be increased by an individual's lack of skill in establishing priorities and allocating time. Role ambiguity also may be a function of an individual's poor discriminatory powers or unclear information from role partners. Upon returning to school, you may identify many of the preceding types of role stress as applicable to your situation, because role stress is very common during position shifts.

Role strain is the subjective feeling of discomfort (tension, anxiety, frustration) experienced by a role occupant exposed to role stress (Hardy and Conway, 1978, p. 76). Not everyone will experience role strain in the same situation, because the meanings we give to situations and our repertoire of responses vary. For example, one employee may prefer a position with role ambiguity, seeing it as an opportunity to create a role, while another may experience acute role strain because of the lack of clear direction. Nevertheless, the experience of role strain is a signal that something is wrong and signals the need for coping strategies. Although the experience of role strain does trigger attempts to alleviate the discomfort, role strain is a common experience in our complex society. It occurs so often that Goode (1973, p. 104) states that difficulty in meeting role demands is normal, because in general our total role obligations are overdemanding.

A special category of role stress and resulting role strain has been labeled "role shock" by Minkler and Biller (1979). Role shock is experienced as "The tensions and stresses arising from (1) radical discrepancies between ideal or anticipated roles and roles which are actually encountered, or (2) the sudden and significant departure from familiar roles which are either enacted differently in the new situation or replaced altogether by new and unfamiliar roles" (Minkler and Biller, 1979, p. 128). Minkler and Biller argue that role shock is a common experience in the workplace. Students of many professions enter their first job only to find that the work role is not what they expected it would be. Workers changing jobs may also experience role shock when they discover that a role in the new organization is not what it was in the previous organization, with the result that familiar behavior is no longer appropriate.

Role shock may occur other than in the workplace. Some of you may find that returning to school is not what you expected it would be. Others may find that the role of nurse expected in school is different from the role you are familiar and comfortable with. Role shock may be central to your experience upon returning to school.

Coping with Role Stress and Strain

A range of strategies is open to the individual as he strives to strike a better bargain in a given role or role cluster. While the following suggestions are not exhaustive, both social strategies and psychological strategies will be discussed. One must remember, too, that not all strategies are possible or helpful in any given situation of role strain.

The *social strategies* involve altering the structure of the situation, that is, changing the relationships in which one is embedded. These strategies include selecting positions, delegation, extension of role relationships, and role negotiation.

To select a position means that one can choose to engage in or drop a select role. This strategy is not realistic for many of the roles we play, but it is an option for some. There are times when a viable option to role strain is to say "no," to drop a role. "I cannot continue as childbirth educator because I am returning to school."

Role delegation reduces role strain through the process of delegating some of the role responsibilities to another, thereby lessening the role demands felt by an individual. Parents may assign household responsibilities to their adolescent children, for example. This is a very useful strategy for students returning to school, too.

The strategy of extending role relationships is one that frequently catches up with you and backfires. With this strategy, one expands role relations in order to plead these new commitments as an excuse for not fulfilling other obligations one finds undesirable for some reason. The danger is that your role partners will not accept the excuse consistently, so you must meet all demands at least minimally or else deal with dissatisfied role partners. Sometimes expanding one's role relationships facilitates other role demands, as when the in-service educator becomes active in an educators' network and thereby enlarges the pool of acquaintances who may be resources for future educational programs.

Finally, one may use the strategy of role negotiation. Through the process of role making, one can strive for a role bargain with another that is as gratifying and minimally conflicting as possible. Sometimes the limitations on what can be achieved are not set by the two role partners, but by interested third parties. For example, hospital medical staffs have been known to deny privileges to physicians who are perceived as striking unacceptable role bargains with nurses negotiating an expanded role. Such third parties try to influence either or both role partners to change the relationship back toward the group norm.

There are also *psychological strategies* one can use in dealing with role stress. These strategies do not really change the structure of the situation; instead, they change the meaning one attributes to the situation. Three such strategies include compartmentalization, selecting a preferred reference group, and reframing.

Compartmentalization enables you to ignore the inconsistency in your role cluster, because you emphasize whatever role is primary in a specific situation and put conflicting roles out of your mind for the time being. This author found herself using this strategy when she left home to complete a doctoral program. The roles of married woman and doctoral student presented numerous conflicting expectations, especially when the program was too far away to permit completing it while living at home. The conflict was minimized by compartmentalization. While away from home as a doctoral student, she accepted that as the primary role, and all energy went into meeting those obligations. When home, however, she gave priority to the role of married woman: a minimum of school work was carried home and preference was given to activities that husband and wife could do as a couple. Such contingencies as location contribute to the workability of this strategy. The geographically separate locations in which these roles were played certainly facilitated this strategy. Even so, as time went by, the need was felt for integration of these two identities, and opportunities to do this were sought. However, having become comfortable and confident in each role separately, she made the final integration.

One can handle conflicting expectations and evaluations of self by clinging to the perspective of a preferred reference group and dismissing the points of view of others. Your reference group is the group with which you identify and whose norms and values you hold, "that group whose perspective constitutes the frame of reference of the actor" (Shibutani, 1965, p. 563). There is no denying that the world of academia holds different norms and values from the world of work. The world of academia is supposed to provide an arena where the work to be done is the exploration and generation of ideas. All sides of an issue must be examined. It should provide an arena where one can imagine what might be, and not simply teach conformity to what is. The world of work, however, is more action than idea oriented. The person most valued in the world of work can rapidly assess priorities and act in a way that satisfactorily accomplishes the task. Because of the press for action, only those aspects of the situation that your experience has taught you are important are considered, while all other dimensions are selectively ignored. Freidson's discussion of the "clinical mentality" is an example of this problem-oriented focus of the world of work of the practicing physician (Freidson, 1973, Chapter 8).

A nurse comfortable with the action mode of work may not view the opportunity to explore ideas and alternatives as important, but instead may see this as impractical and irrelevant. Furthermore, with this resistance to the task, such a nurse may then do the work of academia poorly and receive negative evaluations from important others in the school setting. We have the ability to assign priorities to our roles, to invest more in some than in others, to selectively attend to or ignore socializing clues and expectations. This nurse could cling to the values of the work reference group even while in the academic role and dismiss as unimportant the messages coming from individuals in the educational setting. Such a strategy may soothe a wounded identity, but it may also result in maintaining a chronic adversary relationship with faculty and classmates or in producing failure in the role of student.

Finally, one can use the strategy of reframing (Watzlawick, Weakland, and Fisch, 1974), that is, changing your definition of the situation. Take the preceding situation. Reframing might change a situation of conflict (when one value system is defined as better than another) to a recognition of *differences*. Reframed, academia and the world of work are just two arenas with different tasks and differing norms and values to facilitate that task. Reframed, there is less need to feel a traitor to your working nurse identity, while critically assessing the nursing role as a student. Research has shown that altering the definition of the situation is important in coping. The meaning we attribute to a situation influences the coping efforts we will use. For example, a study of coping in a sample of middle-aged adults found that situations defined as ones where something constructive could be done or in which more information was needed generated problem-focused coping. Situations defined as ones that had to be accepted or in which the person had to hold back from acting generated emotion-focused coping (Folkman and Lazarus, 1980). Reframing is not always easy to accomplish on your own. It is helped by an openness to the points of view of others.

SUMMARY

Role theory is a perspective with great utility for analyzing the social situations in which we find ourselves. It gives us a way of understanding and coping with the social group pressures we perceive and our feelings about ourselves. If, in fact, dissension and conflict among norms and roles is the usual state of affairs, as Goode (1973, p. 110) believes, then your ability to understand the role stress you experience upon returning to school should serve you in good stead. You should find many opportunities to apply this framework to other areas of your life experience, as well as to the experiences of your clients.

REFERENCES

Cooley, C. H. *Human Nature and the Social Order*. New York: Charles Scribner's Sons, 1902.

Folkman, S., and R. S. Lazarus. "An Analysis of Coping in a Middle-aged Community Sample," *Journal of Health and Social Behavior*, 21 (1980), pp. 219–239.

Freidson, E. *Profession of Medicine*. New York: Dodd, Mead & Co., 1973.

Goode, W. *Explorations in Social Theory*. New York: Oxford University Press, 1973.

Hardy, M., and M. Conway. *Role Theory: Perspectives for Health Professionals*. New York: Appleton-Century-Crofts, 1978.

Holland, R. *Self and Social Context*. New York: St. Martin's Press, Inc., 1977.

Kuhn, M., and T. McPartland. "An Empirical Investigation of Self-attitudes," in *Symbolic Interaction: A Reader in Social Psychology*, ed. J. Manis and B. Meltzer. Boston: Allyn & Bacon, Inc., 1967.

Lofland, J. *Deviance and Identity*. Englewood Cliffs, N.J.: Prentice-Hall, Inc., 1969.

Minkler, M., and R. Biller. "Role Shock: A Tool for Conceptualizing Stresses Accompanying Disruptive Role Transitions," *Human Relations*, 32 (1979), 125–140.

Rose, A. "A Systematic Summary of Symbolic Interaction Theory," in *Conceptual Models for Nursing Practice*, ed. J. Riehl and C. Roy. New York: Appleton-Century-Crofts, 1980.

Shibutani, T. "Reference Groups as Perspectives," *American Journal of Sociology*, 60 (1965), pp. 562–570.

Stryker, S. "Symbolic Interaction as an Approach to Family Research," *Marriage and Family Living*, 21 (1959), pp. 111–119.

Turner, R., "Role-taking: Process versus Conformity," in *Human Behavior and Social Process: An Interactionist Approach*, ed. A. Rose. Boston: Houghton Mifflin Company, 1962.

——. *Family Interaction*. New York: John Wiley & Sons, Inc., 1970.

Watzlawick, P., J. Weakland, and R. Fisch. *Change*. New York: W. W. Norton & Co., Inc., 1974.

PART TWO
THE RETURNING-TO-SCHOOL SYNDROME

5

The First Steps

Donea L. Shane, R.N., M.S.

You've made the momentous decision of choosing a school. You've gotten through the maze of paperwork involved in getting admitted. You've made important contacts on campus and are developing meaningful friendships and relationships with some exciting people. You feel wonderful at this point. You have taken charge of your life and made thoughtful and far-reaching changes that will have a significant impact on your career and your future, and you are feeling optimistic about how easy this returning to school is actually going to be. You are getting started into the classwork, and although it may be a little intimidating, essentially you are confident that you will zip through this degree—maybe making straight A's—without too much effort.

We have a name for this mood. It is called "the honeymoon." We recognize this phase as a specific entity because we have observed educationally mobile nurses experiencing it, year after year after year. We did not know about honeymoon until we observed the end of the honeymoon. It was this change in mood, from the optimistic, enthusiastic, delighted new student to an unhappy, obviously disturbed, experienced student, that stimulated us to look closely at nurses who were returning to school.

Pretend for a moment that you are an instructor in a school of nursing that admits educationally mobile nurses. You know that your program is a good one, that it is squarely within the mainstream of nursing education, and that the faculty is skilled and conscientious. Your school produces fine nurses. Why is it, you ask yourself, that so many students seem unhappy at some point during their school years?

69

THE SEARCH FOR UNDERSTANDING

It was the noticeable, recurring unhappiness of educationally mobile nurse students that prompted the systematic observations and subsequent beginning formulations of the returning-to-school syndrome (RTSS). Over a six year period data from the following sources were gathered:

Confidential Diaries - 309 total

Advisement Interviews - 639

Written critiques of RTSS - 72

Retrospective reviews of "Where are you in RTSS" - 41

Seminar discussions with a total of 87 people for a total of 91 hours.

In addition, a faculty survey was done, and a videotape and learning package on RTSS was created by students involved in the program.

A key data source was the confidential diary kept by each educationally mobile nurse for a portion of a semester each year. The diaries were analyzed for similarities and trends. Observations made by various faculty members were recorded; graduates of the program were contacted and informally interviewed; data gathered during advisement sessions were analyzed. Through the six years of this process, hunches developed concerning the commonalities and patterns of students' experiences were confirmed.

Scientists who study the physical world (for example, astronomers, physicists, chemists) add to their store of knowledge by making very precise *measurements* (they usually speak of these as "observations") under controlled conditions. After many observations of this sort, scientists begin to construct an explanation of the phenomenon being studied. By using statistical means, they move toward *predicting* some event, based on the knowledge gained through the painstaking measurement process. The next step is to *control* events, so that some desired aim can be achieved—guiding a spaceship to Saturn, splitting the atom, or producing nylon.

Those people interested in understanding human behavior in the real world (rather than human behavior in artificial laboratory settings) have a much more difficult task. Controlled conditions, by definition, are not "real." Measuring tools may be very difficult to construct and may seriously interfere with the "realness" of the situation under study. And, in human society, is "control" a worthy aim? Stake (1978) suggests that scientists interested in knowing more about human situations

70

should start with multiple observations made over a long period of time until *understanding* is reached. After that, *expectations* about similar situations can be articulated, with the result being appropriate *action*. The ultimate aim of both physical scientists and behavioral scientists (those who undertake disciplined inquiry leading to an understanding of human experiences in the real world) is the generation of natural *laws*, those bits of knowledge that apparently hold true for all places, all times, and under every imaginable condition.

Our qualitative field study of educationally mobile nurses has led us to an understanding of a process that we expect occurs to some extent to every educationally mobile nurse. Further research is needed to investigate many aspects of the RTSS; certainly we need to understand it better before any definitive action can be taken. We consider the concepts reported here to be a beginning effort in elucidating, defining, naming, and conceptualizing a particular phenomenon.

"Wait! Wait a minute here," you are saying. "How can anyone possibly know what is happening to me?" You are right that the particular details of your experience are unique. The RTSS is a *general* framework that describes similarities in the experiences of educationally mobile nurses. Generalization is a characteristic of most theories about human behavior. Freud, Erikson, and Piaget (just to mention a few well-known theorists) describe in general terms what happens to most people in certain situations. Each individual possesses unique characteristics that cause variations; each situation contains original elements. However, there are enough observable, describable similarities present for patterns to be discerned.

Theories attempt to explain the truth of a situation. But is the truth ever fully and completely known? Our history indicates that the answer to this rather profound question is "no." We use our observations and our fertile imaginations to explain phenomena; then we continually modify our operating theories to come closer to the truth, as further use of the theory or additional investigation reveals that we had originally imperfectly understood aspects of the phenomenon. The "full truth" lies forever just beyond the horizon of our knowledge.

Nothing is so useful as a good theory, however. We all develop theories about everything we do, see, or experience. Human behavior is a constant round of developing informal theories, testing their accuracy, developing strategies to modify predictable outcomes, and evaluating the efficacy of our chosen actions. The study reported here is no different. It was developed from observations, and it will be used by people as long as it is helpful in some way. If it is not helpful, it will be modified or rejected. At this time, it is as close to the truth of the situation as careful observations and thoughtful analysis can take us; it represents the second level of theory building, the factor-relating level (Dickoff, James, and Wiedenbach, 1968).

CULTURE SHOCK, FUTURE SHOCK, CHANGE SHOCK, AND ROLE SHOCK

The RTSS is similar to another theory called *culture shock*. Culture shock was first described by Oberg (1960) and Nostrand (1966) and has come to be known as an expression of anxiety. This anxiety can range from mild irritability to panic and crisis; it is precipitated by the loss of the familiar signs and symbols of social interaction of a person's "home" culture when the person becomes immersed in a new and unknown culture. Toffler (1970) used culture shock as a basis for a theory he developed called *future shock*. Future shock is culture shock in one's home culture brought on by rapid change and the subsequent loss of familiar guideposts to behavior.

Within nursing, Kramer (1974) has utilized culture shock to develop her theory known as *reality shock*. Reality shock occurs when the newly graduated nurse enters the world of work. Behavior that won the student high grades and positive comments from faculty members may, in the work setting, earn the newly employed nurse only negative consequences.

Thus several theorists have utilized culture shock. While culture shock describes feelings of alienations and distress, Adler (1975) makes the point that it also provides opportunities for self-development, cultural learning, and personal growth if it is viewed as a positive transitional experience, leading to greater personal awareness and effectiveness. We believe the same is true for educationally mobile nurses experiencing the returning-to-school syndrome. Even though we have used the term "syndrome" in the title, we do not view the RTSS as a disease or a pathological state. It is a normal, predictable outcome of enrolling nurses in nursing programs in institutions of higher education. It can provide an opportunity for meaningful growth if it is handled with sensitivity, understanding, and responsible concern.

At another level of analysis, we can conceptualize all the "shock" situations as *role shock*. Minkler and Biller (1979) have suggested that role shock occurs whenever a person who has learned a particular role is put in a situation in which the familiar role actions are no longer effective or adequate. The concept of role shock is congruent with our observations of people experiencing the returning-to-school syndrome.

THE RETURNING-TO-SCHOOL
SYNDROME: AN OVERVIEW

Definition   The returning-to-school syndrome is a series of positive and negative emotional states experienced to some degree by all educationally mobile nurses enrolled in nursing programs. These emotions arise from role differences encountered in the nursing world the students know best and the world of the educational program that they enter.

We describe RTSS as a series of stages. However, an individual nurse may not proceed through these phases in a linear fashion. The usual progression is an irregular one, with relapses, detours, and expressways through certain stages.

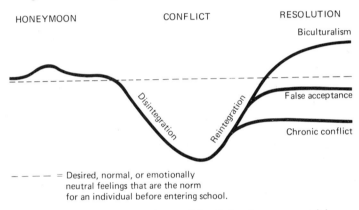

HONEYMOON   CONFLICT   RESOLUTION

Biculturalism

Disintegration   Reintegration

False acceptance

Chronic conflict

− − − − = Desired, normal, or emotionally neutral feelings that are the norm for an individual before entering school.

Figure 5-1   The Returning-to-School Syndrome: a model.

Figure 5-1 illustrates the major stages of the returning-to-school syndrome. The heavy black line charts emotional ups and downs. An upward slope indicates positive feelings, and a downward slope indicates negative feelings. The dashed horizontal line denotes emotionally neutral feelings, the norm for an individual.

The three major stages of RTSS (honeymoon, conflict, and resolution) are unequal in length and intensity. Honeymoon tends to be relatively short and mild. Conflict can be prolonged and intense. Resolution varies greatly from individual to individual in duration, intensity, and final outcome.

Phase I   *Honeymoon* is a delightful time characterized by happy feelings. Even though it is an enjoyable, pleasant experience, it offers little opportunity for dramatic growth and change. One senses overtones of a rather childlike naiveté in people experiencing honeymoon.

Phase II *Conflict* is the most dramatic of the RTSS stages and is unquestionably the source of some educators' idea that educationally mobile nurses are "difficult to work with." Conflict is subdivided into two parts: disintegration and reintegration.

Disintegration is painful and potentially harmful. It is characterized by anxiety that is turned inward, resulting in a variety of negative states, which may include depression, withdrawal from social contacts, and sullenness. It can be easily overlooked by friends, family, and faculty.

Reintegration is also painful and potentially harmful, and its effects may spread to those around the educationally mobile nurse, especially to faculty. Reintegration is based upon a rejection of the current educational program, and the hallmark emotion is frustrated anger. These feelings may be expressed as hostility, which can be directed toward significant people occupying various roles within the educational setting. Family and friends occasionally become the targets of hostile action.

Altough dramatic emotional outbursts may occur during reintegration, it is in some ways a healthier state than disintegration. Strong emotions are being expressed rather than repressed to cause debilitating depression.

Phase III *Resolution* is a critically important stage. It can take a variety of forms.

Biculturalism is the most positive resolution for the returning-to-school syndrome. The bicultural educationally mobile nurse feels good inside, feels good about the first educational experience in nursing, and feels good about the present program. The bicultural nurse clearly sees the differences in values and role expectations of the various roles that have been explored and experienced, and assigns values to each of them. Self-confident and eager to grow and change both professionally and personally, the bicultural nurse is a sophisticated and cosmopolitan citizen of several worlds in nursing who appreciates each of the worlds for its own intrinsic value and its value to the profession of nursing and to society as a whole.

False acceptance is one of the less positive resolutions to RTSS. It is characterized by self-deception and game playing. In false acceptance, the educationally mobile nurse deludes self and possibly faculty into thinking that biculturalism has been reached. But, in fact, large amounts of precious energy are being spent on nonproductive emotions. This less than completely honest expression of feelings means that the educationally mobile nurse has not genuinely accepted the worth or validity of the program now being experienced. The new role has not been genuinely "grown into." Unfortunately, teaching people about RTSS may increase the likelihood of their becoming victims of false acceptance.

Chronic conflict is the least desirable resolution to RTSS. Nurses stuck in chronic conflict spend their time being angry. Although they may not drop out of school, they are unable to recognize the value and worth of the new role being presented to them in their present educational program. They continue to squander irreplaceable time and energy on defense or attack; therefore, relatively little growth and change can occur.

Oscillation is the term used to describe the movement of an individual from one resolution to another, usually one that has already been experienced to some extent. It is not actually a stage of RTSS as such, but is rather a process that can occur at any time. Some frequently observed oscillations are from biculturalism to false acceptance, from false acceptance to chronic hostility, and from biculturalism to chronic hostility. An oscillation (most frequently a regression to a more negative state) usually occurs because of some unusual stressor, such as failure on an exam, an illness at home, or an unfortunate interchange with a faculty member. Oscillations are common occurrences and represent the dynamic, changeable nature of RTSS. They are reversible. See Figure 5-2.

OSCILLATIONS

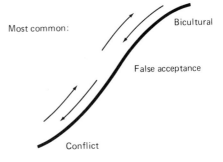

Most common:

Bicultural

False acceptance

Conflict

Figure 5-2 Oscillations. The most common oscillations are from biculturalism to false acceptance, from false acceptance to conflict, and from biculturalism to conflict. All are reversible.

Denial

Since the beginning formulations of RTSS were developed, we have occasionally worked with educationally mobile nurses who vehemently deny that RTSS applies to them, even though they are clearly displaying some of the signs and symptoms of RTSS. Such nurses seem to resent being labeled and categorized, or even being understood. One nursing educator has reported that junior students (typically deep in the throes of anger and anxiety) tend to reject the notion that RTSS exists, where-as senior students confirm that the RTSS theory accurately reflects, in a conceptual way, their experiences. Only additional years of experience in teaching nurses about RTSS will shed light on this phenomenon.

Preview

Each of the phases of RTSS will be thoroughly explored in the remainder of Part II. Our overview has introduced you to the major concepts and terms utilized in describing the returning-to-school syndrome. As you read the remainder of Part II, compare your experiences with those described. Do you see generalizations that help you understand yourself and your situation more clearly? Are you able to stand back from an uncomfortable situation and analyze it by using RTSS concepts? We hope the answer to these questions is a resounding "yes!"

STAGE I: HONEYMOON

The following is a series of interchanges between a nurse who is exploring the possibilities of returning to school and the advisor in the nursing school. The interchanges were chosen because they are typical and based on the author's participation and observation in over 600 such sessions.

Session One

Educationally mobile nurse (EMN):   I'm thinking about getting my degree, so I'm here to find out how much you folks will take of my previous work, how long it'll take me, how much I have to do over . . . that sort of thing.

Nursing faculty advisor (NFA):   Great. Here's our program.
[*Explains details of requirements.*]
We do a course-by-course review of your college transcript for any previous college-level work you have done, then make a decision on which courses the university can accept.
[*Together they review the transcript. According to this particular university's rules and policies, this student can transfer the equivalent of approximately one semester's work.*]

EMN: [*miffed*]
Do you mean to tell me that for three years in a diploma school, I'm going to get only one semester's worth of credit!

NFA: [*attempting to pour oil in troubled waters*]
We know you have lots of experience and prior education, which unfortunately are not in the form of college credits. This university, as a policy, does not have a mechanism for giving credit for life experience, nor can we accept credits earned outside a university system—the diploma school you went to. But, we *do* have a mechanism for *validating* what you know.
[*Explains opportunities for challenging courses, taking CLEP exams, and so on.*)
And we do have these ways of facilitating your progress.
[*Explains accelerating mechanisms devised for educationally mobile nurses.*]
So, it looks like it would take you about four to five semesters to finish the requirements for this degree.

EMN: [*excitedly*]
Wow! This is really different than I thought it would be. You hear so many awful things about this school. I thought I was going to have to start all over again. This sounds like I could really do it! You know, getting this degree is something I've wanted to do for a long time. Tell me again, exactly what I have to do, and where I start.

Session Two

[*EMN has taken some courses, and is making good progress, but has not yet taken a clinical nursing course.*]

EMN: I just had to come tell you that I'm really enjoying the sociology course. The chemistry course just about did me in, but I got a B! That's better than I did the first time I took chemistry. I feel I'm really getting back into the swing of studying again. It isn't so different from when I was in school before.

NFA: Are you having any particular difficulties?

EMN: Well, I've had to make some adjustments at home, and my work schedule needed some rearranging, but my head nurse was really understanding about that. All in all, things are going better than I had expected.

NFA: Let's see, you're taking the Introduction to Professional Nursing course, aren't you? How's that going?

EMN: Well, so far there has been some pretty wild theoretical junk in it. But, you know, I just study that to pass the exams. The history of nursing is all stuff I've heard before, I just had forgotten some of it. I think my diploma school actually did a better job teaching it than this course is doing, but it is pretty much the same.

NFA: How do you like being on campus?

EMN: Once I learned where to find a parking space, it's gotten easier! Actually, I love it. I've got several friends that I carpool with, and we usually eat lunch together and study together. I like being out of the hospital for a part of each week too—the campus is so different that I find it sort of relaxing in some ways. But I'm looking forward to starting the clinical courses. I want to get this degree over as soon as possible, and get on with my life.

Session Three

[EMN has just started taking a nursing course that involves clinical practice.]

EMN: *[passionately]*
I can't believe this is happening to me! Things were going so well, but now it's just awful. I hate this course, I hate the instructors, and I'm so upset all the time I can hardly function! I thought I was going to get through this school without any hassle, but I guess it's going to happen to me too.

NFA: *[knowing that the honeymoon is truly over]*
Tell me what's happening.

EMN: It seems that everything I do is wrong! I study the wrong things and get so-so grades. I thought I'd get A's without any studying—after all, I've been a nurse for eight years. I've always gotten good evaluations from my employer. Plus I disagree with so much of the lecture and reading material. It just isn't the way we do things at work. I just want to scream— this isn't really the way it is! And I'm so *nervous* in clinical. My hand actually shakes sometimes. I'm so afraid that I'm going to flunk! I just don't know what the instructor wants, and she's always asking me why I'm doing things, following me around. It really rattles me.
                                                [Wrings hands, starts crying.]
I guess I'm just not the nurse I thought I was.

These reconstructed interchanges were chosen to illustrate the typical themes we have observed occurring during the honeymoon phase of RTSS and its rather dramatic ending. More explicitly, these themes are as follows:

An initial wariness about returning to school is overcome. The nurse has investigated the options and has made the critical decision of where to go to school. Energy is thrown into making the decision the right one. Disquieting reports about other peoples' problems with returning to school are discounted.

Perceptually, the nurse focuses on similarities between this school experience and prior educational experiences. Values, procedures, and content, for instance, are seen as being essentially similar. Differences in educational techniques, content, or values are not perceived as being especially important, if they are noted at all.

During honeymoon, the educationally mobile nurse's identity as a nurse is not being threatened. At this point in RTSS, students have not been exposed to any experiences that force a questioning of how they, as individuals, play the role of "nurse." Thus, during this phase, one's self-esteem as a nurse remains securely intact; it is not being challenged, and therefore no energy is being put into defending it.

The stresses felt during honeymoon are usually logistical and manageable. These stresses center around how to get registered, how to pay for classes, how to arrange for babysitting, how to manage a work schedule, how to get the washing done this week, how to find time to study. The honeymooning nurse solves these problems more or less efficiently. Each solved problem reinforces the feeling of being an adult who is in control, succeeding in juggling a myriad of worthwhile roles, and moving toward accomplishing an important goal.

The honeymooning nurse's reported reasons for returning to school do not include the expectation that the individual's performance as a nurse will change dramatically. It has been, in our experience, rare for a honeymooning nurse to express anything that would indicate a feeling that there is a need or desire to change as a nurse. Honeymooning nurses feel content and satisfied about their current nursing performance. The words used to convey one's goals for returning to school center around "getting my degree" (curiously enough, few people say "earning my degree," perhaps an indication of the idea that the dues for the degree have already been paid), "getting this over with," or "having to do this." A substantial number of honeymooning nurses clearly articulate their belief that nothing about their nursing performance should, or will, change as a result of returning to school.

Time is a concern. Anyone who knows adults knows that they feel pressured by time—too little time to meet all their responsibilities, too little time to waste it on unimportant things, too little time before life will have slipped by and important things will be left unaccomplished. The honeymooning nurse has an intimation of these feelings and in some ways may express them strongly; but during honeymoon, time pressure rarely becomes panic. Time, during the honeymoon, is a motivator, not a demoralizer.

Not much is known about school. Even though, by definition, an educationally mobile nurse is someone who has already successfully completed a prior nursing program, the typical returning-to-school nurse is unfamiliar with the kind of school now being attended. The L.P.N. attending an A.D.N. program is usually moving from a vocational education background to a junior college setting; the diploma nurse getting a B.S.N. is moving from a hospital setting to a university setting; the associate degree graduate is moving into an upper-division college or university, which may be quite different from the lower-division setting first experienced. The associate degree graduate probably has the most experience with the new educational setting, and there may be many diploma or L.P.N. graduates who have had prior college experience. However, it is our observation that educationally mobile nurses may have unrealistic expectations or misinformation about what the new setting is like. A common misconception is that someone else will do all the choosing of courses and registering for a student (just as it was in a diploma school).

Happiness predominates. During honeymoon, educationally mobile nurses are dealing with stresses, solving problems, feeling content with themselves as nurses, succeeding in their classes, learning how to survive in a somewhat alien environment, and for the most part enjoying the whole experience. It is a wonderful time.

End of the Honeymoon

From our data, it is very easy to pinpoint the end of the honeymoon. It occurs during the first course in which the educationally mobile nurse's *self-image as a nurse* is on the line, that is, the first clinical nursing course. During this course, the student is confronted with performing as a nurse. There is no hiding behind a recitation of experiences, no substituting one's dazzling resume for performance, no escaping the inevitable evaluation. It is terribly intimidating, and the anxiety that is generated by this process catapults the nurse from honeymoon into phase II of the returning-to-school syndrome: conflict.

George Mead's ideas about the relationships between the roles one assumes and one's identity (Hardy and Conway, 1978, pp. 48–50) can be utilized to analyze and understand the end-of-the-honeymoon events. If we accept the premise that the self is defined by the collection of roles one assumes, any threat to one of the roles is a threat to the self. The degree of threat is probably proportional to the degree in which the definition of self depends upon a certain role. It is our observation that most nurses define themselves as "nurse" (to the exclusion of other possible definitions of self) in a major way. This is probably a function of the very thorough socialization processes that occur in the basic nursing education program and in the subsequent socialization processes that are encountered in the work world. Because of the enormous importance of one's own definition of one's self as a nurse, even a tiny pinprick in the substance of that definition *feels* like a stab wound to the person experiencing it.

On many occasions we have observed individuals having difficulty in their "student" role. For instance, a statistics course causes conceptual difficulties for some nurses. A chemistry course seems to be beyond some people's ability to memorize organic formulas. The first nursing theory course may stimulate some intellectual or philosophical questioning. None of these difficulties, however, are usually enough to end the honeymoon. It is when nurses are forced to display their performances *as nurses* that the honeymoon ends. Nurses can fail a math course with more grace and resiliency than they can tolerate a lukewarm evaluation in their first nursing clinical course.

Try this experiment: Ask some nurses who have successfully completed degrees *outside nursing* (it does not matter in which fields) whether they felt worried, threatened, or upset about their nursing performance as a result of their returning-to-school experiences. The answers will probably be "no." They might give examples of how their nursing performance was *enhanced*: "I learned a lot about health teaching that I'm now able to implement," or "the course I took in economics helped me understand hospital budgeting better," or "the anthropological perspective helps me be more sensitive to culturally different patients." Learning about economics, health education, and anthropology touches only tangentially one's definition of oneself as a nurse. Thus we come to this paradoxical, unexpected thought: Nurses studying nursing may at some points in the educational process *feel* worse (more threatened, unhappy, anxious, tense) than nurses studying other fields. This may have a great deal to do with the continuing popularity of degrees established for nurses that include no nursing courses. Nurses enrolled in such programs are never evaluated as nurses, the faculty in such programs rarely has detailed or experiential knowledge of what nurses do. Thus one's "nursing" identity is never challenged or threatened.

There is no evidence that nursing faculty members deliberately wish to threaten or frighten their experienced nurse–students. In fact, most faculty members are sensitive to the interpersonal and intrapersonal issues present in returning to school. The threat to one's self-concept simply rises out of the situation of returning to a nursing school. Although there are undoubtedly individual variations in what triggers a threat, how threatened a particular individual might feel, or how rapidly an individual can recover from a threat, our data indicate that the *risk* for a self-concept threat experience is high during the first clinical course.

There is little evidence that nurses entering a higher-level nursing school *anticipate* that their self-concept as nurses might be under any kind of risk. On the contrary, during the honeymoon stage nurses express their sense of self-confidence and belief in themselves as being fine nurses. The typical self-report is that "I'm a good nurse; I'm not going to change much as a nurse because I'm successful right now; I know so much about nursing already that there is really very little I'll have to learn; I anticipate that getting this nursing degree will be pretty easy." The feelings of threat to one's self-concept as a nurse, then, are even more shocking when they occur because they are so unexpected.

What triggers threats to nurses' self-concept? In general, we have observed two main classifications of triggers: (1) evaluative signals (usually informal) from faculty to nurse–students that may or may not be misperceived, and (2) messages that force an examination of long-held values.

Evaluative signals can be very subtle: a look, an offhand comment, a sincerely meant suggestion that is misinterpreted to be a criticism. In other cases, the evaluative signals are being deliberately sent by the faculty member because some part of the nurse–student's performance is considered to be under par. In either case, the effect of the evaluative signal may be exaggerated by the nurse–student. The pinprick (sent) feels like a stab wound (the perception) to the nurse–student's self-concept.

Messages that force a values examination usually are more direct. In baccalaureate nursing schools, for instance, there is an emphasis upon health maintenance and health promotion. Many nurses have not been exposed to the idea that nurses should play a part in health; their values center around the nurse's role in illness. Thus there may be a tendency to discredit or devalue the time and energy put into educating nurses about health promotion. When it becomes clear to the nurse that the school genuinely values this emphasis, the nurse's own values about health promotion must then be reexamined.

Growth and Change

Nursing educators believe that they are in the business of changing every student's behavior so that it matches a preconceived ideal nursing role that will be necessary *in the future* (Bevis, 1978, p. 52). Their behavior is governed by this belief. Educationally mobile nurses believe that they are enacting an important, worthwhile nursing role already; their behavior also is shaped by this belief. To the extent that there is divergence in the two conceptualizations (the ideal future nursing role as conceived by the nursing educators and the actual role displayed by the educationally mobile nurse), there is area for damage to the self-concept of the student. If, in fact, the educationally mobile nurse *does* know and can demonstrate through behavior the ideal role that the nursing educators are attempting to shape, then the nurse–student will be reinforced; no damage to the self-concept as a nurse will have been done, and relatively little change will occur. If the nurse–student is unable to demonstrate the behavior of the ideal role a school is committed to teaching, predictably the nursing educators will attempt to mold and shape that nurse's behavior until it more closely resembles the ideal behavior. The molding and shaping are done by using every technique known to teachers, some of which can be perceived by the nurse–students as threats to their self-concepts. Changing behavior, however, is the very essence of education; it is also the process by which humans grow and mature.

REFERENCES

Adler, P. "The Transitional Experience: An Alternative View of Culture Shock," *Journal of Humanistic Psychology*, 15, no. 4 (1975), p. 13.

Bevis, E. O. *Curriculum Building in Nursing*, 2nd ed. St. Louis: C. V. Mosby Company, 1978.

Dickoff, J., P. James, and E. Wiedenbach. "Theory in a Practice Discipline. Part II," *Nursing Research*, 17, no. 6 (1968), pp. 545–554.

Hardy, M. E., and M. E. Conway, *Role Theory: Perspectives for Health Professionals*. New York: Appleton-Century-Crofts, 1978.

Kramer, M. *Reality Shock*. St. Louis: C. V. Mosby Company, 1974.

Minkler, M., and R. P. Biller. "Role Shock: A Tool for Conceptualizing Stresses Accompanying Disruptive Role Transitions, *Human Relations*, 32 (1979), pp. 125–140.

Norstrand, H. "Describing and Teaching the Sociocultural Context of a Foreign Language and Literature," *Trends in Language Teaching*, ed. A. Valdman. New York: McGraw-Hill Book Co., 1966.

Oberg, K. "Cultural Shock Adjustment to New Cultural Environments," *Practical Anthropology*, 7, no. 4 (1960), pp. 177–182.

Stake, R. E. "The Case Study Method in Social Inquiry," *Educational Research*, 7, no. 2 (1978), pp. 5–8.

Toffler, A. *Future Shock*. New York: Random House, Inc., 1970.

6
Conflict

Donea L. Shane, R.N., M.S.

OVERVIEW OF THE
CONFLICT STAGE

After the honeymoon ends (as it always does), conflict occurs. Conflict is the stage of RTSS that has always been attention getting. It is fraught with drama, pain, high feeling levels, sound and fury. It also contains the energy for further growth and sets the stage for better things to come.

The conflict stage of the returning-to-school syndrome is comprised of two phases: the distintegration phase and the reintegration phase. During both phases the educationally mobile nurse is feeling some disturbing, turbulent emotions. The difference between the two phases lies in the expression of these feelings. During disintegration, the negative feelings of anxiety and anger are turned inward toward the self. During reintegration, the negative feelings are expressed outwardly, with the anger being directed toward others.

The educationally mobile nurse may experience conflict with beliefs, with currently held roles in the family or work setting, with prior knowledge, with instructors, and with instructional techniques. The potential for conflict exists whenever role changes occur. Looking at role change intellectually, however, is far different from experiencing it personally. Just as people reading statistics about auto accidents do not believe it can happen to them, educationally mobile nurses reading about RTSS find it difficult to believe this will ever affect them personally.

84

The first time I read the article [on RTSS] I thought that much of what you described was exaggerated and those feelings would never be applicable to me. Surely I would never have such feelings of hostility toward a program I was anxiously waiting to enter. I began to get an idea of what you were saying when I took a course this summer, but I really felt RTSS at the beginning of [the first clinical course], just as you predicted. I reread the article then, and it made more sense to me. Suddenly I could identify with those feelings you described. I think I am still in conflict at this point . . . but at other times I feel I can indeed cope . . ..

R.N., married, around thirty.
Quote from RTSS critique.

Conflict with Beliefs

Three beliefs, commonly held by educationally mobile nurses, appear to be important in the development of the conflict stage of RTSS:

1. This new program is *no different* from the program I completed previously.
2. I *know* all there is that is important to know about nursing already.
3. I can *do* nursing better than graduates of this program before I begin study in the program.

The "no difference" belief usually is composed of two subbeliefs: (1) the content and educational processes of the new and the old program will be essentially the same, and (2) the scope of practice in each program will be similar. Holders of this belief seem to be saying that there is no difference between the roles of the L.P.N. and the R.N., no difference in the scope of practice of the diploma graduate and the B.S.N.

The "know it already" belief assumes that the new academic program will be teaching to current practice in nursing, that the educationally mobile nurse has kept current in all aspects of nursing, and that all material presented in the original program has been retained in the brain of the nurse.

The "superior doer" belief is usually based upon the belief-holder's current nursing role compared with the performance of new graduates in the *belief-holder's role.* For instance, the educationally mobile nurse who happens to be an L.P.N. enrolled in a B.S.N. program may enter the program convinced that he is a better nurse, at that point, than the graduates of the B.S.N. program. However, he is probably making a judgment about *how good an L.P.N.* the B.S.N. graduates he has observed appear to be. He uses his own role as the basis of comparison for the role of the graduates of the higher educational level.

Essentially, these beliefs add up to the conviction that nothing will change as a result of experiencing the new program. The nursing role will not change, the knowledge base will stay essentially the same, maybe with some minor updating, and the nursing performance (which is already very good) certainly cannot be improved much.

The present licensing system for registered nurses reinforces the beliefs that nothing much will change. As long as graduates of two-, three-, and four-year programs take the same state board examinations for licensure, they have reasonable grounds to assume that there are similarities in the structure, content, and function of the various educational programs. However, there is some beginning evidence that L.P.N.s frequently hold the three beliefs even though the licensing exams for L.P.N.s differ from those for R.N.s. Obviously, the separation of the nursing profession into several truly distinct levels has not occurred in the minds of most nurses. Not until reality in terms of salary, roles, and licensure reflects distinct, genuine, and consistent reinforcement of the differences that do exist will educationally mobile nurses abandon their beliefs that there are no differences.

Conflict with Family Roles

Undoubtedly a major source of stress to educationally mobile nurses arises from the changes in their home and family roles that they experience when they return to school. Finding time to perform all their roles is a serious problem for returning-to-school nurses, and it is a theme that is frequently expressed in their diaries.

> The first tests are taken and it's down to the long haul. Some of the anxiety is gone. What remains is the reality of the amount of work involved. Between my five classes, I don't have a spare minute. I keep telling myself that it's only four months of time. The thing that worries me a little is that I have time to read my material only once. If I'm really tired or get distracted, that's just tough, because that's all the time there is. I hope nobody in my family gets sick, breaks anything or generally falls apart until Christmas.
>
> R.N., mother, around thirty.
> Quote from diary.

> Tuesday. Tonight I am feeling overwhelmed. Everything seems so confusing. I kept telling myself how I was going to really keep up with everything and do a good job. Now I have feelings that I don't know if I can do it. I keep thinking and hoping that when I get all my things organized and buy all my books, I will feel a lot better. Right at this minute I feel terrible. Tomorrow I have to drive home and attend a funeral so when I get back I will really start in on everything.

Thursday. Tonight I am going to sit down and separate and organize all of my materials and maybe start reading. Things are getting a little more clear and I am not so confused. Thank goodness there are no labs this week. I am very tired and I can't seem to get caught up on my rest. I am also very irritable and cranky with my children. I am beginning to have very negative feelings about putting so much time into myself and my work and not spending enough time with them. I am really beginning to think that I've taken on too much by going back to school and also being a good mother to my children.

> R.N., late twenties.
> Quote from diary.

Sometimes families are slow to recognize the new role the educational mobile nurse has assumed.

I felt disappointed this evening. The kids monopolized the conversation with tales of their first days of school and no one even wanted to know how my first day had gone. I should be used to it by now. I'll always be in the mommy role to my children—they just don't see me as a student despite all the studying they see me do.

> R.N., married, three children, inactive.
> Quote from diary.

Conflict with Work Roles: Realism versus Idealism

Nurses who continue working full or part time while they attend school sometimes feel conflict between the role of student and that of worker.

There is knowledge to be obtained in school and I am trying to get as much out of it as possible. There are times, though, when I feel school is presenting me with the idealistic picture of nursing and work is such that those ideals cannot come true. This is when I feel hostile at the school . . . because they are presenting me with ideals I can't live up to. It is very frustrating, yet I do wish the ideals could become true. So in my work I live up to them as much as I think I can realistically in the situation I am in.

> R.N., ICU nurse, twenties, unmarried.
> Quote from diary.

I [felt] the conflict of realism versus idealism. This at first astounded me. I was not prepared for this. As the semester went on I began to realize that the idealism wasn't so bad. For if one accepts the reality of a situation there is little possibility for a change. If one has the idealism, one has a better chance of incorporating change. Idealism has brought to me the view of different theories and ideas.

> R.N., assistant head nurse, thirties.
> Quote from diary.

I have experienced a little of a "guilt phenomenon." I do see where this program is trying to guide and lead the future of nursing and I do want to see it get there. But I have felt guilty about this at times, thinking "is this too idealistic?" What about the reality of working as an RN in the hospital? Or, am I being a traitor to my fellow workers, or to myself as I have been functioning in that role for two and a half years?

R.N., active, single.
Quote from diary.

One of the reasons I returned to school was my discontent with some of the values of the real world of hospital nursing. On the other hand, I have problems with some of the nit-picky idealism of the school, as well as an inconsistency and vagueness of objectives to be met. I don't really want to return to the old but am really hassled by the stress of the new. Sometimes I toy with the idea of a lateral arabesque into another profession. I seem to vascillate between idealism and nihilism (all of nursing is a farce) with acute episodes of depression and hostility interspersed with real enthusiasm when the pressure to achieve lifts enough for me to enjoy what I'm learning.

R.N., mid-thirties.
Quote from diary.

So far I have felt that the presented picture of a hospital staff nurse to be unimportant and more dependent than other roles. Perhaps this is because the level we are studying deals with the healthy coping client. But it does stir a little anger in me that the job I have been doing is not even given credit—at least not yet . . . . For me the conflict exists not because I feel I'm being told I'm not a good nurse as much as I'm told "What you've been doing isn't really important."

R.N., mid-twenties, single, ICU nurse.

Conflict between Prior Knowledge and New Knowledge

One of the major difficulties confronting schools of nursing that accept experienced nurses is the wide variation in knowledge and skills these students bring to the learning process. Sitting in the same classroom may be a nurse with twenty years of experience following a diploma education, one with no experience who has just graduated from an associate degree school, and an inactive nurse who has not worked in fifteen years. There may also be a large group of brand-new nursing students who may know little about nursing as yet, but who have solid backgrounds in the sciences, humanities, and social studies. Imagine the lecturer's dilemma. There is a good chance that every sentence uttered will be both beyond some people's understanding and boringly redundant for others.

Redundant material, that is, hearing or reading about something you already know, is a source of conflict to some adult students who feel intensely pressured to finish school quickly. They desperately (and quite understandably) want to spend their time and money on nothing but material that they want and need to know. The problem is that the definition of what constitutes new material is different for each individual. Various approaches to individualizing content to be learned have been tried, but the final answer to this problem has not been found or implemented.

> Going back to the building-block theory of the RN to BSN educational system, one discovers that for the most part, it is more of a "pretend you don't know anything and start all over" system. I don't think I can fully convey the boredom, frustration and anger one feels after plowing through one-hundred and fifty pages of required reading only to realize that this is information that you have been successfully utilizing for years. There's a sense of being ripped off, of participating in an elaborate farce of Bettering Yourself.
>
> R.N., married, ICU nurse.

> By my third week in classes, I began to experience actual physical nervous tension, not because of anxiety, but because of frustration and increasing anger as I realized that my expectations for learning were not being met. Although repetition has been cited as the "mother of all learning," I began to experience increasing anger and apathy at the repetition of material not at all new to me. Soon, I began to feel depressed and caught in a trap because I knew there was so much I needed and wanted to learn, but I was faced with the reality that it was not happening for me and would not happen during this semester. My experience with conflict this semester has been due to my expectations of learning new material based on my experience last year, but finding out that this was not the case. I have found this semester to be a waste of time for me academically. I have been feeling angry about this because time is very precious to me since I have been given this time by my Community to study.
>
> R.N., late twenties, experienced staff nurse,
> from semester summary of RTSS.

An educationally mobile nurse in the *same classes* wrote this in her diary:

> I started reading the required materials and I am amazed at how much of the terms, etc., I am unfamiliar with. I'm beginning to see why RN students are required to take [these courses]. It seems to me that anyone would be lost in the wealth of information presented on assessment and nursing process unless he graduated very recently or has been working in a setting where physical assessment, etc. is actively practiced by nurses.
>
> R.N., thirties.

I do feel that the RN student does have an extra problem. We all come from so many different backgrounds but all possessing some (or is it a lot?) of basic knowledge. This knowledge often interferes with learning such as a repetitious lecture that lulls me into a false sense of security where I ignore the "new" information, or a lecture in which my pre-knowledge conflicts with the information given, and my mind rejects the new information because of habit.

> R.N., forties, inactive recently.
> Quote from diary.

I think I've made a personal discovery. When all is going well for me I can really get behind the baccalaureate emphasis on community, validation, four dimensional considerations, etc., but when I begin to feel insecure I tend to revert to a diploma type. I tend to want definite physical problems to deal with, a more structured situation to operate within, and I have a strong urge to rely on intuition.

> R.N., forties.
> Quote from diary.

Conflict with Instructors

The personal relationship between the educationally mobile nurse and the faculty members in a school of nursing can range from marvelous to awful. Furthermore, a particular instructor may be able to establish a very positive relationship with one group of educationally mobile nurses, but be bitterly resented by another group. An instructor who is feared and avoided at the beginning of a semester may be viewed as a fun-loving, supportive, all-right kind of person by the end of the semester. At this stage of our research, we can draw no conclusions about student-faculty relationships, other than that they are obviously an important source of conflict to educationally mobile nurses (apparent from the frequent mention of instructor–student encounters recorded in diaries) and that student feelings about individual instructors may change dramatically over time.

My first attempt to seek guidance from a clinical instructor left me feeling patronized, humiliated and railroaded. Today's clinical was <u>optional</u>. I chose to go because my client is depressed and withdrawn, and I felt that short, more frequent contacts were in order. I did not, however, feel the need to attend post-conference, just this once, because I planned to spend five to fifteen minutes with the client then thirty to sixty minutes reviewing the chart . . . . I was also riding with someone else who was not going to see her client and did not want to attend post-conference. Oh well, skip the gory details. Thanks to an understanding chauffeur I went to post-conference because I knew that instructor could fail me or give me an incomplete, and her only response would be to quote the rules. That's not all. My approach to my client was criticized without asking for my rationale, or even hardly allowing me to get a word in edgewise so I could volunteer my rationale. And, in my eagerness to try to communicate my good intentions (i.e., just because I'm wearing a white uniform doesn't mean I think I know it all), I let her bully me into taking an approach to my client with which I was not comfortable. I'm pretty upset with myself for that. I vascillate between anger and despair. I need help with this client, but I need help in developing my approach. I got the distinct feeling that my learning of nursing behavior was not nearly so important as my learning who was boss today. I really tried to approach all faculty members in a friendly, supportive, open-minded way. There is only one of the three clinical instructors whom I respect, because I perceive that she respects me. She is not a pushover. She has high standards. But she is wise enough to know that if she explains her rationale I will listen and respond to the best of my ability. That is a far cry from sermonizing on my so-called lack of ability to "distinguish between a social relationship and a professional one" (which is what this instructor did, among other things). I had really wanted to share my thinking about my client with the [respected] instructor, but she was busy with another student and the other instructor was obviously available. So as not to offend, I opened right up to this other instructor, and BAM!

Now, I would like to go to this troublesome faculty member and try to establish some kind of rapport, but I'm afraid. There are, after all, some people in life who aren't approachable and trying with them only comes to grief. I need this BSN so I can get on to graduate school so I can do the thing I love (teach) for a few years before I collect social security. However, I'm in danger of learning that obsequiousness is the road to professionalism.

I am used to being treated this way by physicians and health care bureaucrats; how sad that such behavior should come from someone who I would have liked to regard as a role model. Fat chance now. How ironic that some of the most rigid (and therefore technical?) behavior should come from those who have never been afflicted with a "technical base."

[Following week] . . . Sometimes I wish I didn't take life so seriously. In the long run, who cares? And what will it matter five years from now? It will only matter if I flunk clinical and have to take an extra semester out of my life to complete the program. I am expected to obtain a comprehensive health history (a new and awkward skill for me) from a depressed, withdrawn, barely communicative person, and the feedback I get from my "resource person" tempts me to use the client for a role model.

[Next week] . . . Second clinical experience was 200% better. Had an opportunity to consult with [respected] faculty member and got some support for my observations and approaches, as well as constructive advice on new approaches. The [problematic] instructor seemed less uptight about rules and logistics. At one point I noticed the respected instructor surrounded by a group of students (RN and generic) while the other two teachers sat a short distance away by themselves. So I approached them with a brief logistical question: do I need to go to two post-conferences if I go to clinical two days per week? I would classify the response I got as "problem solving" rather than judgmental. It was gratifying. I generally feel much better, but regret the energy I wasted being upset over the first week of clinical and wish I could have avoided it somehow. I spent two to three hours just catharting into this diary!

R.N., thirties,
experienced nursing service administrator,
from diary.

This week was extremely high pressured, intense and exhausting. By the time Thursday rolled around I felt like I had gone through eight days instead of four. Clinical was interesting and in fact enjoyable—a definite break from the routine of reading and videos. I fail to understand why professors feel that they must pressure students so much. Having been through it before, I object to the pushing and prodding. I also feel at times that they treat us like children: fill in your computer cards darker, etc. I just felt extremely negative this past week. Hopefully next week will improve. I've started running again which should balance things out a bit.

R.N., twenties, staff nurse.
Quote from diary.

In clinical; three instructors. Number one sounds like, "This is my/the problem, conflict, goal or rationale in dealing with your questions, request or need." This implies: You are capable of understanding, using good judgment, making intelligent decision. The effect on me: Good self-image, promotes learning, will work hard.

Number two sounds like, "You will perform in this specific fashion. My way is the only way. Why didn't you do thus and so?" This implies: You are not capable of understanding, using good judgment, making intelligent decisions. There is something basically wrong with you. I expect you to be a thorn in my side. The effect on me: Stifles learning. Better off not to risk asking questions, for advice or for help. Volunteer nothing. Maintain non-contributory low profile. Avoid! Avoid!

Number three sounds like, "Don't rock the boat. How could you even consider doing that? I may not be comfortable or know the answer but I can talk about it at length and with (inappropriate?) humor." This implies: You are somehow a threat. The effect on me: Overwhelmed. May receive incomplete or unsatisfying answers. Feel defensive. Insecure learning situation. Proceed with CAUTION.

R.N., forties,
inactive for several years.
Quote from diary.

Conflict with Teaching Styles

Anxiety sometimes arises from the ambiguity of a situation. In academia, an instructor may deliberately plan an experience in which the student must make major decisions, such as where and when to do a project, what client to work with, what topic to study in depth, as a way of helping the student become more self-directive and independent. Furthermore, at some levels of education, particularly at the graduate level, it is very common practice for the students in the class to have the major responsibility for developing the content and method of presentation. However, educationally mobile nurses who have experienced earlier programs that were very concretely planned, with no opportunity for the student to make decisions about the learning process, may feel anxiety when confronted with ambiguity in the new program.

> I was feeling pretty good about the way things were going this week until my clinical group finally met with our instructor. And now, as a result of that meeting, I am once more anxiety ridden. The plan for our group of twelve students is totally different from any one else's. Instead of going to each clinical setting for a four week block of time, we are to combine the settings and use our own judgment in choosing which area we want to go to each week. The instructor will be at the geriatric home on Wednesdays and the elementary school on Fridays, and we are to go to whichever setting we feel will be most beneficial to the goals we have to achieve in the class.
>
> I can see the theory and logic behind this idea, but it is rather frightening to have to worry about whether I have selected the correct setting every week and whether I am accomplishing the things I need to do in order to pass the clinical. It is self paced, and I don't know that I need that sort of hassle right now.
>
> R.N., thirties, married, inactive.

Stereotyping

People enmeshed in the throes of culture shock sometimes attempt to cope with their feelings by stereotyping the natives of the country in which they are residing. All the natives seem to look alike; their skills and attitudes seem to be identical. The culture-shocked visitor cannot perceive individual differences and uniquenesses. Conversely, the natives of a country may have difficulty sorting out the tourists and visitors as unique individuals. The tourists come through in groups, they do not stay long, and the host country typically responds to them as interchangeable units in order to cope with them efficiently and cost effectively.

We have observed a similar phenomenon occurring in the conflict stage of RTSS. There is a tendency for students to stereotype faculty, and a similar tendency for faculty to stereotype students.

The stereotyped view of a faculty member, as seen by overstressed students, is that of an ivory-tower dweller who is not really aware of the everyday problems in nursing, and perhaps not able to make it in the real world of nursing. It is rare for students to see the overstressed situation of the typical nursing faculty member: a woman who frequently is attempting to juggle the roles of mother, wife, student, and full-time worker in the academic setting.

An insightful view of the stereotypes faculty hold of R.N. students has been provided by a former R.N. student in a baccalaureate program, who now teaches in a nursing program. Here are her comments:

> After completing the first four years of a five year BSN program, I left to marry and moved 3000 miles away. Financial circumstances necessitated transfer to a diploma program. I had been an excellent student in the BSN program. I had begun an honor code on that university campus and had been selected by faculty to be the student representative on the faculty committee to begin an honor society chapter on that campus. Five years later I returned and although an RN, I was readmitted as a generic student and began my senior year, much as if I had just taken a leave of absence. As an RN student in that senior year I was a straight "A" student and graduated "with honors" from the university. But unfortunately, I was also now an RN student, and suffered (in silence) insult after insult from faculty as I lived with the stereotypes.

> **Stereotype 1: R.N.s Know Nothing about Families**   Overnight I became someone who knew nothing about families generally, although the faculty member with whom I was working (i.e. who was following my family caseload) told me I was doing very well. The public health nurse I worked with was very pleased that I had made assessments she had previously overlooked, and had made progress with families, previously considered to be hopelessly crisis prone. I wasn't a wonder student, I simply had more time to spend with these families than the public health nurse had. But I continued to hear from other faculty members that as an RN student I just had no understanding of "family." It was amazing that they never considered that I had the same background as my basic generic classmates. It was of course tainted with five years of practice in critical care as an RN.

> **Stereotype 2: R.N.s Really Like to do Tasks**   As an RN student, I was fascinated by the concept of bonding. However, in the postpartum area, I was given twice the caseload as my classmates because I was an RN and could "give baths and make beds faster than my classmates." It mattered little to my instructor that my plan had been to work with two heavily sedated primiparious mothers who, twenty-four hours after delivery, still hadn't realized that they had delivered.

> **Stereotype 3: R.N. Students Know Nothing about Community**   In the last quarter of this long year when my young classmates were choosing an area of concentration, of course mine was chosen for me. Naturally, because I was an RN student, I had to be in public health because "as an RN student, I knew nothing about community." In the preceding quarter I had made an

"A" in community nursing and had just presented an in depth study of an inner city area which faculty had evaluated as being "excellent."

> Quote from a letter, by a 31-year-old former ICU nurse,
> presently an assistant professor of nursing and a
> doctoral student in nursing.

Stereotyping is a coping mechanism for those who use it. It reduces the need to spend energy on figuring out who an individual really is, how that person wants or needs to be treated, or in modifying one's own behavior in response to an individual. Stereotyping permits the utilization of standardized approaches to groups of individuals. For that reason, it will probably continue to be used by both faculty and students. However, our data indicate that stereotyping is a source of anger and frustration.

DISINTEGRATION

Anxiety

During the honeymoon stage, the educationally mobile nurse has been focusing on how similar the new educational program is compared to the original nursing program experience. The perceived similarities are very comforting and tend to reinforce the feeling that pursuing the new degree will be relatively easy and nonthreatening. The end of the honeymoon usually begins with a shifting of attention to the *differences* between the new program and the previous nursing education experience. These differences may include unfamiliar teaching methods, differences in content, value differences, even different definitions of what constitutes nursing practice. The nurse sometimes engages in an internal monologue that goes something like this: "This is not the way I have been operating. Is it possible that I have been practicing wrong? Is it possible that I'm not the good nurse I thought I was? Is it possible that I'm a bad nurse?"

May (1950) says anxiety is "apprehension cued off by a threat to some value which the individual holds essential to his existence as a personality." An educationally mobile nurse has spent years establishing a personal identity as a nurse. It is easy to understand the source of anxiety when this hard-won identity is threatened in some way.

Every diary and every interview we have reviewed has revealed anxiety. People differ in how much anxiety they feel, as well as how long they feel it, and they express it in many different ways. However, anxiety is such a pervasive characteristic of educationally mobile nurses that we have come to view it as a predictable, normal phenomenon.

The anxiety began the week before school started. The anticipated written examination and return demonstration had my anxiety level up. My anxiety was enhanced more by "grapevine" communication that a certain instructor was "very rough" with students. The day of the return demonstration I fell further apart when this so-called "rough instructor" became my observer for the return demonstration.

I came out of the session in a daze, but relieved. The instructor was terrific! She may have been "picky," but I concluded she was truly interested in the fact that I grasp the theory and principles of the subject matter. She appeared to me to be precise, and to make sure all the things she offered stayed in my gray matter.

> R.N., late thirties, married,
> over ten years experience.
> Quote from diary.

And I thought I'd been tired before. Must be that old devil anxiety! Today, the first Tuesday, I've experienced so many emotions—frustration, optimism, pessimism and even anger. I think my anxiety about having enough time to study coupled with the general confusion and necessary schedule change really did a job on my objectivity today. I know I can master the material—I just don't quite know how yet.

Wednesday evening: I'm a wreck. I have determined that this is the worst I will feel and the greatest anxiety I will suffer for the entire semester! Life is too short. I'm grateful to have the proficiency demonstration over with. To think I have practiced in a clinical setting with some degree of competence.

> R.N., mid-thirties, married, children.
> Quote from diary.

The proficiency exam was today. I really felt that I was a student nurse all over again. I can't believe I felt so awkward doing procedures I have performed over and over again. Part of it was having to consciously think about what I was doing, part of it was being observed. Part of it was knowing that you always haven't done things exactly by the book. Part of it was knowing that I have adapted to the reality of nursing as it is and now I need to adapt to the non-reality of the ideal way. But yet I believe that nursing, as it is, needs to be changed. Another whole facet is that I was being told I was not accepted as an RN at face value, but had to prove myself.

> R.N., mid-twenties, nurse practitioner.
> Quote from diary.

I couldn't sleep last night and my stomach is doing flip flops this morning. I haven't felt this anxious in years. I wish I knew if I passed the written test. What if I get to school, ready to take the [clinical] proficiency test, and the instructor sends me home because I failed the written test! I keep telling myself that it really won't matter if I do fail because I won't be out anything—but I know my pride will be crushed.

[Later] I can't believe I passed the proficiency test! It wasn't as difficult as I had anticipated but I was certainly nervous throughout. Kris [another RN student] and I were so relieved to be finished we went out for lunch and a stiff drink. It's nice to have someone to commiserate with. In retrospect, I think one of the reasons I felt so nervous about taking the proficiency exam is the feeling that it was testing my ability to be a good nurse. I mean, if I can't pass the most basic of nursing skills, what am I doing calling myself an RN? I felt like my vocation was on the line, so to speak. No wonder I felt so anxious.

> R.N., early thirties, married.
> Quote from diary.

Anxiety can be behaviorally expressed in a number of ways. How one handles anxiety is a function of one's background, personality, previous experiences with anxiety, self-esteem, physical health, the perceived degree of threat, and one's sense of poise, to name just a few of the variables present. It has been our experience that the anxiety felt during the return to school is situational; that is, it occurs in response to specific events and does not become a permanent part of the educationally mobile nurse's personality. Furthermore, we observe wide variations in the degree of emotional response to a situation. Our data convince us that much of the behavior displayed by educationally mobile nurses in the conflict stage of RTSS is generated by anxiety.

Anger and Depression

Two students, sitting side by side in a classroom, are confronted with a situation that appears to have identical impact on them. One student responds, "That really upsets me," feels uncomfortable for a time, then moves on to another issue. The second student cries, "I am infuriated! I'd like to bury this place." It is possible that the second student may take action to do so. We have no tools to measure the degree of anger felt by each of these students; thus we do not know if they are feeling the same amount of anger. We can observe, however, that they are *expressing* their feelings in different ways.

Roberts (1978, p. 198) says,

Anger can be viewed as a derivative of anxiety. Incorporated in the feeling of anxiety is a sense of powerlessness. Thomas (1970) identifies how anger follows a social order of events beginning with anxiety. First, one perceives the anxiety-producing situation as something that can or should be managed through overpowering thoughts and/or actions such as fighting, conquering, or subtly opposing. Next, one blunts or avoids it by transforming the energy created by anxiety into thoughts and/or actions designed to control or disguise one's own feelings and/or to overpower a situation or another person. Individuals under stress situations can accumulate only so much energy before it must be channeled constructively or destructively. The excess energy can take the form of hostility or anger . . . .. Anger that is turned inward can force the [person] into depression.

Depression, usually relatively brief and reversible, has been reported by educationally mobile nurses.

> Last year I felt as though I was held responsible for more material than I could ever possible remember, let alone apply. This was especially true of [the growth and development course]. And I thought [the present level] would be the same as having <u>four</u> classes just like the growth and development course. And on top of that I would have to spend x number of hours in labs and clinical whether I needed it or not. Come to think of it, I have been more or less depressed for <u>nearly a year</u> just anticipating [this year].
>
> R.N., early thirties,
> former nurse administrator in small rural hospital.
> Quote from diary.

Other emotions reported by educationally mobile nurses going through the disintegration phase of conflict are sleeplessness, lethargy, apathy, withdrawal from social contacts, sadness, excessive fatigue, a feeling of helplessness, a sullenness that is sometimes observed in classrooms, and a loss of control that results in verbal outbursts. Obviously, these feelings and actions can be harmful both emotionally and professionally. Unfortunately, they may seriously impair the nurse's academic performance so that a downward spiral is created: The nurse feels so apathetic that studying is neglected, then tests or papers are poorly done, which makes the nurse feel even worse, which makes the next round of academic tasks even more difficult to perform successfully.

We have found the most useful antidote to disintegration to be ventilation. If nurses are provided the opportunity to express their feelings and are shown that these feelings are predictable, frequently felt by others, and are usually temporary, our experience has been that disintegration is relatively brief and harmless.

A word of warning: disintegration may be easily overlooked by those around the educationally mobile nurse experiencing it. Because the expression of emotions is directed inward toward the self, the nurse may very well suffer in silence.

REINTEGRATION

Anger and Frustration

The nurse in the reintegration phase of conflict rarely suffers in silence. As in culture shock, the basic mechanism at work in reintegration is a rejection of the "new culture," the academic program. This rejection is expressed usually as hostility.

Hostility is the outwardly displayed acts of an inwardly felt frustration and anger. Hostility is a strong word; no one likes to be branded as a hostile person, especially experienced nurses who generally pride themselves on their interpersonal skills, sense of control over their emotions, and poise under stress. Nevertheless, hostility is a term that creeps into discussions about educationally mobile nurses held by nursing educators. The hostility perceived by nursing educators is the observable manifestation of the anger and frustration being felt by the educationally mobile nurse. Unfortunately, hostile acts may provoke anger and frustration within the nursing educators; these feelings may be followed by hostile acts directed toward students. This results in the "civil war phenomenon" occasionally observed in schools of nursing. One side sends messages to provosts and presidents; the other side shoots off rebuttals. One side may suggest a list of terms for peace; the other side, after deliberation, rejects them. One side may divert attention to a minor issue; the other side retaliates by dropping a bombshell on the major battlefield. As in real wars, the outcomes are usually decided politically (not on the rational merits of either position), and everyone loses. Fortunately, this kind of major conflict is rare.

However, the most poignant aspect of major conflicts is that each side evidently feels essentially the same emotions for essentially the same reasons: They are being frustrated by the actions of the other side in their strivings to reach a goal important to their own role expectations. Nursing educators in such situations predictably are attempting to uphold their cherished values and principles; educationally mobile nurses are typically striving for the least anxiety producing, personally satisfying, and role supportive education they can obtain. It is to be hoped that additional research and thought into the processes and content of nursing education will find ways to reconcile these conflict-producing and presently divergent goals.

Adler (1975) sees the expression of hostility and the rejection of the new culture as a positive sign of healthy reconstruction; it is not always easy for nursing educators to view hostility in this light (Cobin, Traben, and Bullough, 1976; Wooley, 1978), which is understandable.

The nursing faculty member is professionally committed to socializing the educationally mobile nurse into the academic culture; the educationally mobile nurse who is reintegrating, however, is (more or less) vigorously rejecting that culture.

Roberts (1978) states that the "fundamental dynamic force behind hostility is frustration" (p. 198). Frustration is a frequently reported feeling among educationally mobile nurses, perhaps because it is more socially acceptable to report being frustrated than to report being hostile or angry. However, if given the opportunity to safely express their feelings, educationally mobile nurses will occasionally identify their feelings as hostility:

> I cannot abide by the content and manner of teaching here. I have not accepted the best of this world and I am clinging to the old ways. I admit this wholeheartedly . . . I've been hostile for three years now. I realized in (my original) nursing school I would need to do this, and it made me angry. I think my hostility is dormant now and only flares up when very upsetting things happen. I've learned that being angry and complaining doesn't change anything, and so I have attempted this term to live with the rules.
>
> R.N., recent diploma graduate,
> from a paper, "Where Are You in RTSS?"

> I find myself hostile against certain members of the faculty and, in general, hostile against the program. I find that I have many complaints against the program, yet I understand the need for the degree and will value it when I have achieved it. In fact it means everything to me just now.
>
> R.N., recent A.D.N. graduate,
> from a paper, "Where Are You in RTSS?"

> "My moods . . . fluctuate from mild anxiety to panic. I daily consider taking a year off from the program to regain my emotional equilibrium. I am overwhelmed with the volume of material presented and the superfluous quality of it. I detest some of the instructors for their pompous ignorance. I am furious at the grading discrepancies, one instructor giving easy A's while another picks, picks. At the same time, I take comfort in knowing that my tumultous emotions are not unusual and that if I can (and I will!!) get through this that I will see my emotional responses are not completely valid and are the expressions of my high anxiety.
>
> R.N., twenties, ICU experience,
> from a paper, "Where Are You in the RTSS?"

When a person is going through culture shock (see Oberg, 1960), one common sign of the reintegration phase is blaming the foreign culture for all the suffer's ills. We observe the same phenomenon in the returning to school syndrome.

The educationally mobile nurse (while in the throes of the reintegration phase) projects academic difficulties onto the academic program itself. The following are examples.

"I got a poor grade on that test because the questions were badly written." (The test had been given three years in a row, had been item-analyzed three times, and had an excellent history of identifying students' strengths and weaknesses.)

"I'm getting a C out of this course because the observations are ridiculous and I will not waste my precious time doing them." (Ignoring some of the requirements for a course usually has a negative impact on the final grade.)

"I felt good about this program when things were going OK for me, but now I think it is a stinko program, and I'm going to tell everyone how really stinko it is!" This statement was made by an R.N student who had just done rather poorly on an important exam. It clearly illustrates the relationship between the student's feelings toward herself and toward the program. Furthermore, the statement hints at retaliation. The student's image of herself has been wounded, and she is bent on hurting the program in turn. Such is the genesis of hostility. (Incidentally, the student quoted here went on to finish the program very successfully, with a high grade-point average. Whether she spread word about the "stinko" program is unknown, but fairly unlikely.)

For the instructors, advisors, family, peers, and friends surrounding the educationally mobile nurse who is in reintegration, it is important to recognize that many complaints about "the program" may be absolutely valid. Experienced educationally mobile nurses, returning to school as expert clinicians, may very well point out the inaccuracies and obsoleteness of exams. Each complaint about a program must be carefully evaluated on its own merits. Charges of unfairness, improper procedures, inaccurate data, or ambiguous questions must be thoroughly investigated and dealt with reasonably. However, it is also important to realize that the reintegrating educationally mobile nurse may harbor feelings about the program that are related to the perceptions of the grade-point average being earned: good grades produce good feelings and few complaints; poor grades produce poor feelings and many complaints.

When Americans move to a foreign country, it is not uncommon to find them clustered together in a particular neighborhood. Similarly, people who emigrate from other countries to America may be found grouped together within cities, in Little Italy's or Chinatowns, for example. A parallel occurs occasionally among reintegrating educationally mobile nurses. The angry, frustrated students tend to clump together for the same reasons the immigrants from China clump together: It is very comforting to be around people who share your cultural orientation, your values, and your beliefs about a situation. (Of course, one could make the point that immigrants to America are walled off from the major culture deliberately, for the more sinister reasons of prejudice and exploitation. We have not detected such a parallel occurring among student populations.) Nevertheless, the angriest students within a group tend to gravitate toward each other, it seems, probably for the very understandable reasons of mutual support and affirmation of their viewpoints.

Other students may become impatient with the amount of complaining done by the typical reintegrating student, especially those who have worked through their own feelings, are perhaps more objective, or have reached a later stage of RTSS:

> I'm tired of complaining and hearing other people bitching about things. I've decided to either comply and start adjusting to things or I won't get through it. At this point, complaining and griping don't do much other than take energy away from constructive purposes. I feel that if I do stay open minded, I will learn from the classes and labs many things related to healthy people which I hadn't considered as a part of nursing.
>
> R.N., mid-twenties, staff nurse.
> Quote from diary.

The Ultimate Hostile Act

When conflict becomes too painful, when resources cannot be found either internally or externally for working through the feelings of conflict, when there seems to be no letup to the stress, and when the student comes to the conclusion (accurate or inaccurate) that the payment extracted for returning to school is not likely to be worth the ultimate rewards, the student performs the ultimate hostile act: dropping out of school.

Dropping out is usually preceded by feelings of hopelessness and the conviction that there is no other choice to be made. It may be done gently, sadly, and politely or angrily, with slamming doors, red faces, and dramatic announcements.

We do not consider dropping out a true resolution to the conflict stage of RTSS. We do consider it suicide. It is a deliberate act designed to end one's life as a student. There may be an unconscious hope that those left in the environment will feel a little guilty when the dropout is gone. Perhaps they will; many will feel the tragedy inherent in good dreams gone awry. The real tragedy is that conflict stage dropout need not occur. Dropouts due to family moves, finances, illness, or a hundred other reasons, including flunking out, are usually not preventable. Conflict stage dropouts occur because the people involved let them occur.

The major preventatives are (1) understanding and (2) choices. An understanding of the stresses the student in the conflict stage is experiencing seems to be very therapeutic; the understanding listener may be another student, a family member, an instructor, or an advisor. The potential dropout's story should be carefully heard. The next crucial step is to help the potential dropout to see the choices available. Every situation can be dealt with in many different ways; dropping out is only the poorest of a number of ways of handling the situation.

WHO IS RESPONSIBLE
FOR CONFLICT

Because the potential for harm exists in the conflict stage, it is understandable that some people raise the question, just whose fault is this, anyway? Is it the fault of ivory-tower educators and accrediting agencies who have structured programs that unintentionally become painful for some people? Is it the fault of naive nurses who are stuck in intellectual ruts, to whom growth, change, and new ideas are anathema? Is it the fault of the profession of nursing, which has surely been growing and changing, but which has suffered from a lack of clear vision on what changes are needed, and how changes should be made? Is it the fault of those other groups within the health services that have long exerted control over nursing: medicine, hospital administration, regulatory agencies, or third-party payors?

If this were a multiple-choice quiz, the most popular answers would probably be "All of the above" and "None of the above." That is probably the most accurate way to answer this question, too. The responsibility for conflict is a shared one. One group does not have a monopoly on the responsibility for this complex situation, and thus the preventative for conflict (if one exists) cannot arise from one group only.

Perhaps there should be no preventative for conflict. It is entirely possible that the conflict stage is a necessary part of role change and that it is especially severe in educationally mobile nurses because they have assumed their original nursing role so thoroughly and completely. If they are to grow into a new role (and we firmly believe that growth, change, and new roles are as democratically American as the flag), perhaps conflict is essential.

We do not have answers to these questions at this time. Research into the *necessity* for conflict has not been done. Our observations, however, convince us that it grows naturally out of the mix of elements present in nursing at this time.

By definition, the conflict stage is the time during which nurse–students feel the worst; fortunately, the conflict stage is self-limiting. Even though troublesome elements in the situation may not change, people begin feeling better or they begin behaving differently. The diaries of people in conflict generally reflect a tendency toward some resolution about two to four weeks after the initial plunge into this stage. However, it is also true that the feelings of conflict can recur; typically a recurrence happens because of a blow to the student's self-concept. Some examples: a poor evaluation, a grade lower than one hoped to achieve, a critical remark made about a clinical performance.

Conflict is predictable. Every diary submitted to us shows some evidence of conflict as we have described it in this chapter. However, there is a wide variance in the degree to which people appear to be suffering, and there are variations in the length of time people experience feelings of conflict.

Almost every one survives! Good news! Our data show that people survive the conflict stage. In fact, out of the subsample of people whose diaries are directly quoted in this chapter, *all* successfully completed the degree program in which they were enrolled.

As part of our data collection, we studied a group of RNs who were enrolled in the nursing program during the fourth year of the RTSS study. Exactly fifty RNs were enrolled in the program during the Fall semester. We checked to see what had happened to those fifty RN students by the beginning of the sixth year of the study. Out of the fifty students: thirty-three graduated; ten were actively progressing (four people in this group had failed one challenge exam, two people had had babies, one person failed a prerequisite course, and three people were part-time students who were deliberately progressing slowly); four dropped out before entering the upper division courses; two transferred to other colleges or universities; one person was counseled out of the program for academic failures. These data point up the strong motivation seen in educationally mobile nurses to complete a program.

In the next chapter, we will describe the various ways in which people resolve their "Conflict Stage" feelings. The final chapter of Part 2 will give you some strategies for coping with conflict and other RTSS stages.

REFERENCES

Adler, P. S. "The Transitional Experience: An Alternative View of Culture Shock," *Journal of Humanistic Psychology*, 15, no. 4 (1975), p. 13.

Cobin, J., W. Traber, and B. Bullough. "A Five-level Articulated Program," *Nursing Outlook*, 24, no. 5 (1976), pp. 309–312.

May, R. *The Meaning of Anxiety*. New York: Ronald Press Company, 1950.

Oberg, K. "Cultural Shock Adjustments to New Cultural Environments," *Practical Anthropology*, 7, no. 4 (1960), pp. 177–182.

Roberts, S. L. *Behavioral Concepts and Nursing Throughout the Life Span*. Englewood Cliffs, N.J.: Prentice-Hall, Inc., 1978.

Thomas, M. "Anger: A Tool for Developing Self-awareness," *American Journal of Nursing*, 70 (December 1970), p. 2587.

Wooley, A. "From R.N. to B.S.N.: Faculty Perceptions," *Nursing Outlook*, 26, no. 2 (1978), 103–108.

7
Resolutions of RTSS

Donea L. Shane, R.N., M.S.

RESOLUTIONS TO THE CONFLICT STAGE

Roberts (1978) states, "There are several factors which lead to feelings of hostility. These include frustration, loss of self-esteem, or unfulfilled needs of status and prestige." Returning to school seems to generate these feelings in many students; many returning students seem to stimulate these feelings in instructors. Thus, the conflict state of RTSS is characterized by deeply felt emotions; the expression of these feelings may affect surrounding people, such as families, co-workers, and peers.

As scary and traumatic as the conflict stage can be, it is self-limiting. The energy generated by high anxiety levels must be converted into other forms. The intensity of feelings demands resolution.

We have identified three resolutions to RTSS:

1. *Chronic conflict is a maladaptive resolution.* In this resolution, relatively little energy is expended on growth and change, while major amounts of energy go into continued anger, hostility, and frustration. The chronic conflictor may burn down to apathy.

2. *False acceptance is a marginally adaptive resolution.* In this resolution, the educationally mobile nurse uses precious energy to smother and disguise negative emotions. The false acceptor copes, but does not flourish.

3. *Biculturalism is the most positive resolution.* Energy is effi-

106

ciently channeled into growth-producing behaviors. Used in this context, biculturalism is defined as the ability to be as comfortable and effective in the school culture as in the original nursing culture that an individual has experienced.

Oscillations

A prominent feature of the resolution stage of RTSS is the movement of an individual back into a phase that has been experienced previously. This dynamic, moving quality of the resolution stage we have named *oscillation*. Like Grandmother's electric fan, which first cooled the east side of the room, then turned to the west side, the educationally mobile nurse may move from a hard-won false acceptance back into a painful chronic hostility. The stimulus for such movement is usually something in the academic environment: an incident, an interpersonal exchange, a disappointing performance on an important assignment or examination. Occasionally, an oscillation from a positive resolution stage to a more negative stage may occur because of a stimulus arising outside the academic setting, but this is relatively rare in our observation.

When asked to comment on the RTSS theory, an educationally mobile nurse made this statement:

> The types of resolutions, false acceptance, chronic hostility, and biculturalism are aptly described. I don't believe they are static states however; more likely, the student/nurse continuously bounces back and forth depending on the particular rotation, perceived benefit of the course of study, and the attitude of the instructor at that time.
>
> R.N., late twenties.
> From a paper entitled, "Critique of RTSS."

> At the present time, I believe I'm leaning toward biculturalism, realizing that I have learned a lot and that there is much to be gained by the direction I take from here. At the same time, I feel that I will maintain a little cloak of false acceptance which I shall throw around my shoulders from time to time.
>
> R.N., forties.
> Quote from a paper, "Where Are You in RTSS?"

CHRONIC CONFLICT

Chronic conflict is a maladaptive resolution to the conflict stage of RTSS. As the name implies, it is an extension of the angry, frustrated feelings encountered during the conflict stage that lasts for an extended period. The boundaries between the acute conflict stage and chronic conflict are very hazy, but it should be suspected in any person who is feeling angry and frustrated far longer than others in the peer group.

The person in chronic conflict does not drop out of school. In fact, the turbulent emotions may be very motivating. The chronic conflictor declares angrily, "I'll get through this $@#*&&*% school! Nothing will stop me." And nothing does.

But even though the chronic conflictor finishes the program, it may not be a successful experience in terms of growth and change. So much energy is spent defending the original role identity that very little effort is put into genuinely attempting to expand the scope and depth of practice.

As in the conflict stage, the chronic conflictor continues to reject the "new" culture (the present academic program). Roberts (1978, p. 215) notes that the angry person is directing his feelings toward a perceived threat. The threat in this instance is probably the program or its human representatives, the faculty members, which are deliberately trying to change the enrolled student. If the student does not hold the same values as he perceives those connected with the program hold, or if he believes that society does not need the kind of practitioners the program molds, or if he thinks it is just a lackluster program, he is not willing to change in the direction he is being urged to move.

An instructor in the western United States reported the following incident:

> We were discussing infant feeding practices. One of the RN students got very agitated about what I was saying. She kept holding up her hand and making remarks like: "This isn't the way the doctor I work for does it" and "That just isn't how it's done." I made some conciliatory statements indicating that of course there were individual differences in recommended regimens and that some physicians had their own ideas, but the recommendations that I had given the class earlier were the current best thinking on the idea. I even referred her to our textbook—a very recent, well-thought of text—and she still didn't relax. I could see that she left that class still convinced that her ideas were the only right ones, despite other evidence to the contrary. She simply could not entertain the idea that what she had been practicing could be outdated or inaccurate. It was so important for her to cling to the idea that the rest of us were wrong. I kept my eye on that student until she graduated, and I think she never really moved from that attitude. I think she spent all her time here being angry and defensive. For all I know, she still is.
>
> From author's interview files.

For much of the first part of the semester I have to admit I was in chronic hostility. I was bitter at the long hours I was having to put in at school, I was bitter at the financial strain I was causing and I was just plain

pissed off (excuse me) at the ambiguity of it all. It has taken a lot of energy
to come out of it.

> R.N., mid-twenties.
> Quote from a paper entitled, "Where Are You in RTSS?"

Taking [a human growth and development course], I developed all the
symptoms of the conflict stage. I still have hostile feelings toward that course.
I felt as if I were being treated as a child. I'll never get over having to spend
two mornings observing at a nursery school.

> R.N., mid-forties.
> From a paper, "Where Are You in RTSS?"

I have been having lots of sleep disturbances due to finals. I am terribly
tired, and I frequently say something angry. I studied so hard but I did not
feel good about the final in [the physical assessment class]. I just don't know
what my problem is with that class. But, whether my grades are good or bad,
I'm glad to take a break. I'm BURNED OUT.

> L.P.N., recent A.D.N. graduate, early twenties.
> Quote from diary.

FALSE ACCEPTANCE

False acceptance is *a camouflage*. The educationally mobile nurse in
false acceptance is trying terribly hard: trying to be a good student, trying to please instructors, trying not to cause trouble, trying to maintain
a low profile, trying to *look like* the perfect student. Inside, however,
all is not so positive. Deep inside, either consciously or subconsciously,
the false acceptor harbors doubts and anxieties that have not been resolved. Energy is spent in maintaining appearances. Behavior at times is
governed by the feeling that there is a certain game that must be played:
Honest, congruent responses to a situation will not be rewarded.

> So what do I do about this particular crisis? [The diary has described a
> rather humiliating incident with an instructor.] . . . I not only feel I have to
> play games with this faculty member, but I feel there is no way I can win this
> game . . . . It's not really my nursing ego identity that's threatened. I know I
> can be a good technician, but I want to be more. I feel a threat to my adult
> ego-identity. It's not the educational program, its some of the people in it
> who exercise what I perceive to be a careless power over the course of my life
> for next couple of years.

> R.N., staff nurse, thirties, single.
> Quote from diary.

I see the act of hostility totally useless, since it incorporates the use of too much energy being wasted. I accept the fact that there are different ways of doing things and that the way I learned how to do things may be outdated. I no longer find myself stereotyping faculty or blaming them for my weaknesses—I realize that I am the only one who can strengthen them. I understand what is expected of me. I feel I understand the rules and that any energy spent on anger is wasted. But, I still question if what I am doing and the goals that I have set for myself is what is best for me. I still see a large amount of anxiety within me. I continue to have a fear of failure. I expect a great deal from myself and sometimes have difficulty accepting those things that I must do to meet these goals. I see how going to school has affected my family and my work, both positively and negatively. And, I continue to ask myself "Why am I doing this to myself?"

R.N., thirties, pediatric nurse.
From a paper, "Where Are You in RTSS?"

Two thirds of the time, I enjoy school and encountering differing viewpoints. But then, I get thrown back into a game playing situation where I parrot what the instructor wants to hear, instead of learning and growing myself.

R.N., early thirties, staff nurse.
Quote from diary.

I think I am coping fairly well for the most part and my sense of humor is definitely returning. I can laugh at myself again and don't take everything so personally. But my . . . ego image as a nurse is threatened by the upcoming challenges. I had a positive clinical experience (last semester) but I am feeling very anxious and threatened by the challenge clinicals. Also I still find myself questioning the value of the baccalaureate program—perhaps not in general, but this particular program. I feel that in many ways nursing is portrayed in such an idealistic way by the school that they aren't realistically preparing their graduates for the real world of nursing. This is a source of frustration to me and makes me question the value of the program for returning nurses . . . . My goal from the beginning has been to do my best in the program and finish! At this time I feel my goals are still attainable, and I think that by concentrating on those goals, and not concentrating myself at this time about whether or not I like the program, I will be able to achieve biculturalism by the time I graduate.

R.N., thirties.
From a paper, "Where Are You in RTSS?"

In some ways, false acceptance is an iatrogenic condition: the treatment of RTSS (giving information about the condition) may force people to feel that they must camouflage their true feelings. One thoughtful nurse made the following comments when asked to write a critique of RTSS:

I feel that life at any phase must be accepted until each phase is experienced. I did not know how I would feel at thirty until I got there, in spite of what I was told to expect. Now at thirty-six, I can evaluate thirty. I believe that it was stated that in false acceptance one does not believe in the value, worth, or internal validity of the baccalaureate program. I feel that this isn't so abnormal. I will be able to evaluate the baccalaureate program when I go into the nursing profession with one. Also every new experience is evaluated with "pro" and "con" observations. "Bad mouthing" or con expressions as well as pro expressions are as natural as breathing. Perhaps the person expressing con feelings is wasting energy but then so is the interpreter who lets it become a personal attack. In summary, I prefer the false acceptance student to listening to the chronic verbal hostility or frustration of someone who can't get his head screwed on straight.

R.N., single, staff nurse.

Some people reject false acceptance as anything they would personally experience:

Looking back, I reflect on each stage I experienced. Last spring I innocently started with honeymoon and quickly switched to Conflict as fall semester began. The emotions I dealt with consisted of boredom, anger and depression. I find that even though I have begun reintegration, I still feel fairly hostile. This past few weeks I have argued, complained, and fought against the system. I do not feel by any means that I will reach false acceptance. I certainly never keep my emotions bottled up or play games with faculty!

R.N., married, staff nurse.
From a paper, "Where Are You in RTSS?"

I think I am presently . . . less inclined to argue with the requirements of the program—those arguments have obviously not affected the requirements which I completed, and I really have a great deal of demands on my energy resources. This program, like any other program will have its good points and bad points, and since graduation with broadened skills is my objective, that is where my energies will be most productive and where they will be focused.

R.N.,
in paper entitled, "Where Are You in RTSS?"

As several of the nurses quoted have noted, doubts and uncertainties about the educational program exist during false acceptance, but these are not expressed angrily or destructively. These doubts are organized around the following themes:

1. Doubts about the *value* of the educational credential to the enrollee. Is this program really going to help me reach my goals?

2. Doubts about the *worth* of the role being taught in the program. Does society really need people with this degree? Does the health-care system—hospitals, principally—need people who know how to do things the way they are being taught? Is the role a genuine one?

3. Doubts about the *validity* of the particular program. Is this school really a good school? Are the principles and values being taught like those of other high-quality programs of the same type? Are the faculty in this particular school competent? Is this program in the mainstream of nursing education, or have I stumbled into a peculiar, unusual program?

4. Doubts about the student's own *ability* to complete successfully the program. The false acceptor is not thinking about dropping out, but still harbors anxieties about doing well in the academic setting. These anxieties are not nearly as intense as those felt during the conflict stage, but, nevertheless, they exist, they influence behavior, and they consume precious energy.

The following description of the false acceptor was written by an educationally mobile nurse:

> The person who takes false acceptance as their way out might be one who has a "type A personality." They are never satisfied with what they are. Being President is better than being a Vice President. This person usually has worked five to ten years and knows the ins and outs of their institution. They find themselves in a situation where they cannot advance because of bureaucratic policies. They find one way around the block is to get qualified. They go back to school to earn BSNs, MSNs, and if necessary PhDs. They couldn't care less what they are learning. They already know what they need to know. They come to class, learn everything with a closed mind, and maintain the grades to get the degree. Some of these students will excel to a point of being an A student. The instructors know this type of student. In fact, they think most returning nurses are this way. They will try to change them but they will not always succeed. When this student earns his or her degree, he or she will return to their bureaucratic institution and will become bureaucrats themselves.
>
> R.N., former L.P.N., thirties.
> From a paper, "RTSS Critique."

As the semester proceeded, I perceived a large amount of ambiguity built into the program, simply because of difficulty interpreting and understanding what was expected from the behavioral objectives, and from the actual messages received from different instructors. I developed a degree of anxiety I had not known for many years because I could not decide what was expected of me. At that time, I developed a false acceptance type of behavior and tried as hard as I could to in essence say "Teacher, may I?" "Teacher, should I" and "What do *you* think, Teacher?"

R.N., early forties, ICU nurse.
From a semester review of RTSS.

I returned to school mainly because I felt I could be a better qualified nurse if I had a BSN. For six months I worked as an acting head nurse in the emergency room and I just didn't feel qualified. This is what really motivated me to go back to school. I feel that with a broader education and more knowledge, I can go back to be a good head nurse. This is still my goal, and I will continue to work toward it.

The Returning to School Syndrome hit me very hard. I felt that school was going to be real easy because I did well in school before and I felt I was a good efficient nurse. I felt that I would do well because I would be more interested and already had a good background and knowledge base in nursing. I also felt that I would do well because this time I know where I am going and what I want to learn and get out of the program. I was truly in the honeymoon phase.

I began classes feeling very good about everything. I too adored going to school and enjoyed every lecture and was on top of the world. But, slowly but surely, the frustrations, high levels of anxiety, depression, the hopeless feeling, and anger began to creep up on me. My first test results began to show me that I wasn't doing as well as I expected. What made me even more anxious and upset was that the generic students, who never worked as an RN, and never had RN experiences were doing better than me. I realized very fast that even with all my previous knowledge and experience I had to work just as hard as the generic student.

I began to be very angry, because being an RN wasn't helping me at all. I began to ask myself, "What am I doing here?" "Why am I putting myself through this?"

You would think that I'd never been in college before. I felt so frustrated. I felt that the RN behind my name now meant nothing. And even more frustrating: I don't know why I'm not doing well. I study very hard and generally keep up with the readings for lectures. I, too, blame my poor doings on the instructors' bad test. I still don't think I'm projecting and I still think it was a poor test.

At this moment in time I still have feelings of anger and hopelessness. I don't necessarily feel hostile. I have realized that if you are going to make it through this program you have to "play their game." I found that you have to "play the game" even in a work situation to get what you want.

I'm still trying to get the most out of the program, because I not only want a BSN, but I also want more knowledge so that I can go home and take a head nurses position and do a good quality job. I think with this in mind, I am beginning to accept what I have to do to reach my goal.

R.N., twenties.
From a paper, "Where Are You in RTSS?"

The definition of culture shock and the feeling are known to me. I have experienced the feeling several times due to different moves, different situations, that I have been in. It is growth the hard way, but nonetheless, it is growth.

In the nursing area, the honeymoon phase for me lasted only a few days due to the fact that I decided to apply and was accepted in more or less a week's time. During that time I felt I could cope and that if I really disciplined myself, I could succeed. I felt good about the fact that I had taken the "first giant step" as in the kids games. Finally, after all these years, my goal was becoming a reality. Although I was aware of some of the changes in nursing and it's values, I felt I could adjust to the differences. I felt that although my nursing background was not as extensive as I would have liked, it would give me a good basis for building up further nursing skills.

Next came the reality shock, or disillusionment stage. I found that my study habits, retention abilities, and previous knowledge were of little value. I just didn't seem to manage; there was too much to cram, my brain was unreliable—it was failing me—and I was too slow and stupid to continue in this fast-paced world. It was, and still is, a threatening stage in which not only were my nursing abilities being questioned, but my abilities as a person to cope with stress were being put to an acid test. I became disorganized, unable to sleep and irritable (as my family will attest to). I just couldn't believe that all my past experiences couldn't help me through. I had done it before—had had problems with family, teenagers, etc., and I had coped. Had I been an ostrich and buried my head in the sand and not seen what was going on? Had I been unaware of the tremendous changes in nursing and in the whole educational system? What are the expectations and can I live up to them, not just for "their" satisfaction, but for mine? I came back to the nursing area for a degree to further my knowledge so that I can be a better nurse, but this really does not coincide with what I thought I would be doing.

I feel that I am still in a stage of resolution of some type. For all I know, I may be going through a chronic hostility or a false acceptance stage, although I haven't pinpointed that area. Some days I feel good about who I am and what I'm doing and other days I wonder about my coping and managing abilities. I'm becoming a little bit more balanced as I talk to others, and find that almost everyone has a problem to some degree. It is also interesting to know that nursing programs have the same expectations of students, since I have talked to others in different schools.

Perhaps I will feel better, as I progress through the program. I still feel that nursing educators are not as realistic as they could be, and I can see their point in wanting to promote independence, etc., but I do not see any drastic change in nursing immediately. I know my ideas of nursing have changed but there still needs to be more of an actual experiencing of effective changes for the good of clients for me to be a <u>bona fide believer.</u>

R.N., forties,
part-time worker for some years before returning to school.
From paper entitled, "Personal Review of the RTSS."

On the continuum between chronic hostility and biculturalism, I'm veering toward biculturalism. I never even entertained false acceptance because I like to complain loudly too well!

However, this nurse continues,

I'm coping more confidently, knowing the rules and spending psychic energy on growth. Most of the time, I feel my sense of humor is intact. However, I still feel an occasional need to defend my former training and I'm still exhausted on occasion from being so "on guard."

R.N., married, late thirties.

Her comment about being "on guard" is a classic false acceptance feeling.

False acceptance clearly is a coping mechanism that is frequently used by educationally mobile nurses. It is maladaptive to the extent that it blocks the full use of one's potential. However, it is the most positive resolution of RTSS that many people experience. In comparison to chronic conflict, it permits a relatively comfortable completion of a program, and it makes the school environment more pleasant for everyone. There seem to be two major outcomes of false acceptance:

1. Students do not reach their full potential while in school, even though they may be successful in completing the program.
2. Faculty members may be lulled into believing that all is well with students, when in fact only the surfaces are placid.

Biculturalism

The concept of biculturalism (and the word itself) comes directly from culture shock theory. Oberg's original work (1960) on culture shock contains this statement:

In the fourth stage, your adjustment is about as complete as it can be. The visitor now accepts the customs of the country as just another way of living. You operate within the new milieu without a feeling of anxiety although there are moments of strain. Only with a complete grasp of all the cues of social intercourse will this strain disappear. For a long time the individual will understand what the national is saying but he is not always sure what the national means. With a complete adjustment you not only accept the foods, drinks, habits, and customs, but actually begin to enjoy them. When you go on home leave you may even take things back with you and if you leave for good you generally miss the country and the people to whom you have become accustomed. (p. 179)

A somewhat later writer on culture shock, Smalley (1964), says,

> Eventually to some comes a beginning of a sense of humor, a lessening of tension, and the ability to see the funny side of it all. With this of course begins healing and although many strains may remain, recovery is very likely. Once the problems begin to seem funny they are never as overwhelming. Finally, in biculturalism, in a degree of understanding of the new society such that the individual can begin to react in appropriate ways, real victory is obtained. As the new cues are learned and the signs of what is the right thing to do are assimilated, often unconsciously, and as language becomes a strong foundation for the new resident's repertoire of communication media, the bases of tension and hysteria are little by little removed.

In applying these concepts to the returning to school syndrome, we have defined biculturalism as "the ability to be as comfortable and effective in one culture (school) as in another (work)" (Shane, 1980, p. 122). We see it as the most positive resolution to RTSS.

Becoming Bicultural

Some of the most valuable insights we have gained about biculturalism have come from a group of R.N. students who grew up in one culture (they come from several different North American Indian groups) and then had to adjust to the different ways of the dominant American culture when they began their education and nursing careers. Approximately 25 percent of the registered nurses who helped formulate the returning to school syndrome theory are American Indians.

A most articulate American Indian nurse talked about her experiences when she returned to school during a recorded interview:

> I had become a very skillful nurse, I was competent and capable as a nurse and as a physician assistant. My competence was recognized by the employing organization, and so did the Indian community, so I had that support system. My family was very supportive. I knew who I was, my family knew who I was. I came into school, and suddenly I didn't know myself. I didn't know who I was, and I had no support. All I could do was talk about what I could do or what I had done. War stories! I thought: What am I about now? Why do I need to do this?
>
> My response was to become combative, and to try to NOT accept the values that I found in the nursing program. Time was a value; so I flaunted that. I just would not meet deadlines, I would get myself problems because of time. Reading was another value. I read other things—I read so many other things, sociology, psychology, international health, everything but what was assigned by the teachers. But somewhere along the way the challenge business (a requirement of the program) happened, and other nurses started to talk of

it. A new social network was formed! I had not been aware that I was a part of it; the RNs in the group became my support system. They gave me credibility; I was part of that system. With that strength, we told each other war stories. And we found ourselves getting involved with generic students—cuddling and stroking them; so we were doing nursing at that time, telling them to hang in there, things would get better, it just hurts for a little while. I think if that had not happened I would not have been able to exist in this new environment.

I had spent so many years learning skills that were not useful in this new environment. These skills were not required in the new environment, and the skills that were required I did not have. I had a very difficult time getting through. After I had finished, I thought about what I was supposed to have learned, and realized it would have been a good thing if I had learned it.

I left the baccalaureate program with many questions about health, the definition of health, the teaching-learning process. I really have enjoyed the masters program. It is a chance to explore ideas like these, that I had during the baccalaureate program. I'm not fighting any more. I'm trying to learn now. I'm learning basic technical skills that are of value to both cultures (school and work). If you come to my Indian village, I would expect you to learn a few words and a few appropriate behaviors, in order for you to function safely without my having to watch over you all the time. That's what is expected when we come into the academic setting: we expect you to have a few technical skills (reading, writing) which are valued. We expect you to have these appropriate behaviors because we don't want you to get squashed! We can't watch you all the time.

My daughter accompanied me on some business I had one day. I had to visit one of the elders of an Indian village west of here. I talked with the man, asked after his family, and brought up the item of business only after I had paid my respects. We drove back to Santa Fe where I breezed into the supervisor's office. I told him, "It's all set up. Send the letters . . . do this, do that." Afterwards my daughter pointed out to me how differently I had behaved with those two men. With the Indian man I had talked slowly, not brought up business until I had asked after his family, had never made any direct suggestions, had agreed with his ideas, and had used a certain tone of voice. With the supervisor, I had come directly to the point, had not bothered with any social chitchat, had made suggestions on what should be done.

I think my behavior was competent and appropriate in each of these settings. The white man expects certain behavior from me, and the Indian man expects a different kind of behavior. I think that's biculturalism, and I think that is how you become an effective person in two different settings, working with two different people.

R.N., mid-forties, American Indian.
From recorded interview.

I've seen some examples of bicultural behavior among some of the community health nurses who come to my home [Indian] village. They have definite cultural codes that they operate by. They come into the village, they respond to the village needs, the needs of the people, the social activities and religious activities; they're aware of the activities and respond to them appropriately because they have <u>learned</u> the new behaviors.

Say there is a diabetic man in the clinic. He's sick, he's gangrenous, he needs an amputation. The doctor says to Sam, "Come up today, we'll admit you." Sam responds by saying, "I'll come up; I have to go home to get ready." The bicultural nurse understands what Sam is saying. He is saying, "I'm going to go home and have a healing ceremony. I'll be there in four days, when it is over and I'm ready." The clinic nurse may not explain this to the physician, but she knows what will happen and will keep Sam comfortable. She has acted very appropriately and has strengthened her ties with the village people.

The minute the nurse leaves the community and drives back to the city, she is in her own cultural setting. She speaks faster, she writes faster, she meets her guidelines of documenting what she has observed, she communicates with other health professionals, she moves around making referrals. Her behavior is then very appropriate for that setting. The next day she returns to the village, and she is able to change again. Her tone of voice changes, her speech slows down. Again she moves back into this very appropriate behavior she has learned. She may look for positive signs of her acceptance in the village, but there will be no letter of appreciation forthcoming. The fact that people allow her to be there and that people come to her is a sign of her acceptance.

> R.N., forties, Native American.
> From recorded interview.

I believe that I am now well on my way to biculturalism. I have a better understanding of what is expected of me and I am definitely less anxious and tense. I enjoy learning and am getting as much as possible out of the courses. I can recognize my own growth and am able to realize that I will function in a different way when I graduate.

> R.N., mid-thirties.
> From a paper, "Where Are You in RTSS?"

Now that [the first semester of the junior year] has passed and I'm ready for challenging [the second semester of the junior year and the first semester of the senior year] I feel comfortable and think that I'm fairly solidly in biculturalism. [This past semester] was definitely a time of conflict for me, but the combination of a good "changing roles" class, an understanding coordinator—no, I'm not looking for brownie points, I'm speaking honestly—and a cohesive, mutually supportive group of RN student-peers has made me feel very good about myself, the program and the fact that <u>I really am going to get there!</u>

> R.N., mid-twenties.
> From a paper, "Where Are You in RTSS?"

I believe I am in the area of Biculturalism within the Returning to School Syndrome. I see myself on the fringe as yet, because I still continue to experience feelings of depression and frustration. But at least my depression and frustration doesn't stay "around as long." Somehow, knowing that this is a normal cycle I can cope with it better. I believe the Changing Roles class helped me through this first level. The class itself was like a "buffer" and it made things a lot easier to take.

R.N., mid-forties.
From a paper, "Where Are You in RTSS?"

There are times when I feel that I am reaching the biculturalism stage because I've felt good about myself and why I'm back in school. I've been able to see myself in my previous nursing role and now in a much different role as a nurse. I am able to see myself functioning differently, because I know I will have a much more broad knowledge base, and viewpoint. In just going through this past semester, I have picked up a lot of new knowledge that I know I will use when working. At first I was wondering why I did come back, but I now am able to see how much better a nurse I will be when I go home and work again. I'm interested in Emergency Room nursing and the skills I learned in the health assessment class will help me very much. I am able to see myself as an AD graduate and hopefully a BSN graduate.

R.N., twenties.
From a paper, "Where Are You in RTSS?"

The *competency of biculturalism* comes from two sources: (1) the mastery of important skills, and (2) an understanding of the values held by the people who make up each culture. Understanding values does not mean that you must change your own values necessarily, nor does it mean that you must reject all of one culture in order to be effective and competent in another culture. The behavior of the bicultural person becomes acceptable to each culture; the bicultural person does not behave the *same* in each culture, however. When in setting A, with people in culture A, the bicultural person behaves congruently with the people in culture A. When in setting B, the bicultural person acts differently, but again congruent with the people in culture B.

For example, in your workplace you may routinely perform a very abbreviated admission interview on the clients you admit to your unit. The school you are attending has spent hours teaching you a much more elaborate and comprehensive admission interview format. If you are a bicultural nurse, you would become skilled in the school's interview style and demonstrate your competency in it everytime you are given the opportunity. Since your workplace has not demanded more of you, it is possible that your behavior in that setting will not change. However, it is also possible that you may become convinced that a somewhat more complete interview of newly admitted clients would be of benefit; you may take small, but effective steps toward changing the prevailing workplace view of what constitutes an adequate admission interview.

Biculturalism Is Achievable

Our experience has been that most educationally mobile nurses are successful in reducing their feelings of anxiety and in becoming competent and effective students. We observe, with heartwarming regularity, nurses who in the beginning have seemed very uncomfortable in academia becoming confident, good-humored, facile learners. Bicultural nurses, as we are using the term, clearly are spending their precious energy on growth and learning, rather than on nonproductive defensive emotions. They have not abandoned the values learned in the world of work, but have been able to integrate new skills and values learned in academia into their workplace roles. These bicultural nurses have unquestionably expanded their scope of practice in nursing and have developed a broadened perspective on the profession of nursing. They value the educational program in which they are enrolled for its intrinsic worth to them and to the profession of nursing and to society in general. They exhibit a very positive stance toward learning and change. They understand that returning to school not only enhances them as nurses, but has also educated them generally. Their viewpoints, values, attitudes, and skills closely parallel those of other well-educated people in our society.

The Bicultural Nurse as Ambassador

Nurses who are competent and effective in both the workplace and the educational institution should be able to help build bridges between these two entities. Much has been written about the dichotomy between nursing service and nursing education. It is indeed true that nurses who occupy positions in each of these worlds are socialized into different sets of competencies. Nurses who have the ability to be effective in both the school and the workplace will surely, we believe, increase the understanding and rapport between these two vital groups. "Ambassadors" are those nurses who have become so comfortable, skilled, and effective in both the educational setting and the workplace that their acceptance is unquestioned: They belong to each group. Their "belongingness" enables them to deliberately take action that reduces the barriers, misunderstandings, and crossed purposes which occasionally occur between nursing service and nursing education. We firmly believe that the development of a large group of bicultural nurse ambassadors will have a positive effect on all of nursing in the future.

We hope *you* become an effective, competent, and comfortable bicultural nurse ambassador.

REFERENCES

Oberg, K. "Cultural Shock Adjustment to New Cultural Environments," *Practical Anthropology*, 7, no. 4 (1960), pp. 177–182.

Roberts, Sharon L. *Behavioral Concepts and Nursing Throughout the Life Span*. Englewood Cliffs, N.J.: Prentice-Hall, Inc., 1978.

Shane, Donea L. "Returning to School Syndrome," in *Teaching Tomorrow's Nurse: A Nurse Educator Reader*, ed. S. K. Mirin. Wakefield, Mass.: Nursing Resources, Inc., 1980.

Smalley, William A. "Culture Shock, Language Shock, and the Shock of Self-discovery," *Practical Anthropology*, 11, no. 5 (1964), pp. 49–56.

8

Strategies for Coping with RTSS

Donea L. Shane, R.N., M.S.

The preceding chapters of Part II have described the returning-to-school syndrome as we now understand it. RTSS is a process of becoming, not a disease; it includes times of joy, happiness, and accomplishment, as well as moments of despair, tension, and self-doubt. It is a process that predicts changes that begin at the very core of a nurse's self-perception, extend through the roles that a nurse plays in society, and may have an impact on the profession as a whole. RTSS is not a trivial process. We believe it deserves further careful investigation. Additional study may well change some of the findings we have made to date; that is the time-honored method by which knowledge is advanced. Further elucidation of RTSS should include ways to modify the process so that all nurses who return to school will benefit maximally from the experience.

The purpose of this chapter is to help you devise some strategies for successfully coping with your return to school. This advice is gleaned from our contacts with educationally mobile nurses, faculty teaching in nursing programs, and our study of RTSS. We have not done "double-blind" studies on these suggestions in the same manner that new drugs or other kinds of therapeutics are tested. Rather, we offer these pieces of advice in the same spirit that grandmothers offer home remedies: They are comforting, they have grown out of our experience in dealing with problems, and frequently they work.

MAKING THE MOST OF YOUR
KNOWLEDGE OF RTSS

What can you, as a returning-to-school nurse, do with your knowledge of RTSS? Obviously, you should take steps to maximize the good times, while minimizing the bad times. Three key areas to think about are (1) your attitudes, (2) your support systems, and (3) your skills.

Attitudes

The right attitude, it appears to us, can overcome a number of weaknesses in both skills and support systems. Just what is the "right" attitude? *Enthusiasm for learning* is a winning attitude in academia; it conveys your eagerness to grow and change, your happiness about being in academia, your optimism about your future and the future of nursing, and your trust in the professional judgment and wisdom of the nursing educators who have constructed and are implementing the nursing program you are attending. Teachers love to teach enthusiastic learners. The opposite attitude—sullenness, refusal to participate, sarcasm, apathy—may not be fatal in the academic setting, but certainly it will win you few supporters and will do little to increase your comfort in the educational world.

Sometimes it is impossible to manufacture an attitude upon command from your brain. If you are in the clutches of a severe conflict stage downturn, your attitude will not be very enthusiastic. At that point, your knowledge of RTSS should tell you, "I know this is a not uncommon reaction to returning to school; I know it will not last long; I know that this is the outcome of a pretty severe role change and I've expected something like this to happen; I know I will feel better soon." Our experience in teaching people about RTSS is that knowledge of the phenomenon reduces its severity, reduces the length of the conflict stage, and may have some impact on the number of people who reach a genuine, solid, ambassadorial-quality bicultural stage.

Support Systems

Your prime support system when returning to school will be those fellow students who are most nearly like you. If you are an R.N., it will be the other R.N. students at the same point in the curriculum that you are. It is *essential* (we believe) that each returning-to-school nurse obtain

membership in such a group. Enlightened schools of nursing will plan
for such groups by requiring a course that gets you together, by offering
a voluntary study group, or by sponsoring a nurses' club, for example. If
the school you have chosen does not offer such opportunities, take it
upon yourself to develop a formal or informal group of your peers. This
is the age of the peer-group self-help movement, as seen by the number
of groups that help people with problems of alcoholism, obesity, colos-
tomies, partnerless parenthood, and drug abuse. RTSS also appears very
amenable to group help.

The diaries of our study sample of R.N.–students contain numerous
references to the support offered by other R.N.s, and by the Changing
Roles in Nursing class designed to help foster the support-group concept:

> I feel I am entering the resolution phase with brief regressions into mild
> hostility; and acceptance isn't always as honest as I'd like it to be. I am certain
> that I would be in a dead end phase of resolution were it not for the R.N. sup-
> port group.
>
> R.N., forties.
> From a paper, "Where Are You in RTSS?"

> I find that I am really enjoying this semester—finally getting to the ma-
> terial that I've been waiting for, i.e. physical assessment. I see people around
> me getting very anxious concerning different assignments but so far I'm find-
> ing them stimulating. I suppose I'll know if I should have been more anxious
> after I get my grades! I do have a confession—I am enjoying the Changing
> Roles in Nursing class *much* more than I thought I would. I had a very vague
> idea of what the course would be about and I saw it as spending time that
> could be better spent elsewhere. I apologize! It is giving me the support and
> insight I need to keep going. The guest speakers have been great and your in-
> formation and general sense of humor help to keep things in their proper
> perspective. Thanks!
>
> R.N., late twenties, intensive care nurse.
> Quote from diary.

As in any group, informal leaders emerge in groups of returning-to-
school nurses. One uninvestigated aspect of RTSS is how the nature of
the informal leadership of a group of educationally mobile nurses influences the outcomes of RTSS in the group members. For instance,
does the presence of a group leader who is deeply into the conflict stage
of RTSS prolong conflict stage in the group members or maybe sup-
press the emergence of biculturalism? Conversely, does the leadership
of a bicultural ambassador nurture the same RTSS outcome in group
members? We have no answers to these questions, but utilizing what is
now known about group dynamics, it would seem logical that the nature

of group leadership would have some discernible impact on the outcomes of RTSS in the group members. If this is true, perhaps your best strategy in planning for group support that will be most helpful to you in overcoming the negative effects of RTSS is to align yourself with a group whose leader is handling the RTSS transitions competently and effectively. If you are a person who naturally becomes the leader of a group of educationally mobile nurses, think through carefully the impact your own place in RTSS may have on your peers in the group. As an informal leader, your prestige and influence may be an important factor in the outcome of other students' return to school.

Peer-group support can offer many helps to the educationally mobile nurse. You can study together, share triumphs, cry on each others' shoulders, help in managing child care and transportation, share books, photocopy each other's notes, try out new skills on each other, gossip together, laugh together—the list is endless. Holding yourself apart from this source of support is a major mistake and will probably make your RTSS transitions more painful and less positive. Other writers on the many variations of culture shock cited earlier (Oberg, Smalley, Minkler and Biller, Toffler, Kramer) have pointed to the value of group support, and we echo their advice.

Other support systems include families, close friends who are not returning to school, workplace colleagues, and official sources of help such as advisors, counselors, mental health workers, religious workers, and others. These sources vary widely in the amount of help they are able and willing to offer to the individual educationally mobile nurse.

Skills

If you are not a good writer, a shrewd test taker, a skilled memorizer, an elegant conceptual thinker, or a fast reader, it may well be to your advantage to sharpen these skills before you return to school. Perhaps you have previously mastered these skills and all you need at this point is a brief brushing up. Perhaps these are skills you have never mastered, and you need substantial help in becoming reasonably competent in them. Investigate ways you can conveniently add these skills to your list of competencies. They *will* be necessary as you return to school. Your local community may offer several ways for you to sharpen these skills. Self-help books are widely available. Do not fall into the trap of thinking that your present nursing skills alone will be adequate. They are admittedly very important, but so are academic skills. Indeed, academic skills will probably have a larger bearing on your grades (assuming that you are a safe and competent nurse) than your current nursing skills.

SORTING OUT
THE ROLE CHANGES

As you return to school, there are at least two distinct and separate role changes that you will be faced with. It may be helpful to you to clearly sort these out.

The Student Role

Think of this role minus the "nursing" aspect of it. One of the most shocking truths that returning-to-school nurses must face is this: The skills that made you an effective clinical nurse are not necessarily the same skills that will make you a competent student. Competency in the student role is firmly based on intellectual skills: reading, writing, memorizing, analyzing, communicating in a sophisticated way, thinking abstractly and theoretically, and in organizing knowledge in new and untried ways. Competency in the clinical nurse role always revolves around *doing*: performing tasks, organizing the work of others, interacting with clients and families, working under guidelines and policies of an employing institution. Fortunately, there are areas of overlap, and gaining competency in student skills will unquestionably help you perform your clinical nursing role in a new and enhanced manner. As you add additional competencies to your repertoire of skills, you may also become a more flexible and effective person in *all* your many roles.

Usually the more problematic aspects of taking on the student role relate to the powerlessness that most people perceive in the role: lists of objectives to be met (theirs, not yours), readings already chosen for you, activities already planned. Probably the best strategy you can adopt is to play the role of student as it is described by the school to the extent that it is comfortable for you. When you encounter activities or objectives that you find very difficult to live with, figure out what you would be willing to do *as a substitute*. Think through the reasons why your proposed substitution would be especially helpful to you and how the substitution would fit into the general framework of the course. Then present your proposal in a friendly, informal, eager-to-learn manner. Many teachers are open to this sort of negotiation. However, remember that the teacher has as much investment in the role of "teacher" as you have in "nurse." The teacher cannot play the role of "teacher" without reciprocal role partners, those people who are playing the role of "student." So you do not want to behave in a way that negates the teacher's role; your behavior should reinforce the teacher's role, while you negotiate on how you as an individual will play the role of student.

Sometimes educationally mobile nurses find themselves in a class with teachers who were nurse–colleagues in an agency or in some other professional relationship that has already been established. This can cause some confusion and uncertainty about how the teacher–student roles should be played. Probably the most effective strategy for you to adopt if you find yourself in this complex situation is to downplay or de-emphasize prior relationships. They are not relevant to your current student role. The teacher may or may not acknowledge prior relationships, but you would be wise to follow the teacher's lead in this matter: If the teacher makes references to your other relationship you might do so also; if the teacher never mentions any other relationship with you, don't be offended—the teacher is probably attempting to keep your mutually intertwined roles straight, too—but follow that hint and maintain a low profile. The colleague-to-colleague relationship is always different from the teacher–student relationship, and it is unrealistic to expect your prior relationship to continue unchanged in this new situation.

The "Ideal Nurse" Role

The second role change that you will be faced with is that of assuming the behaviors of the "ideal nurse of the future," as defined by the school at this level of education.

Do some careful thinking about what you want to get out of returning to school in terms of your own performance as a nurse. Knowing that nursing educators always attempt to shape ideal performance, can you think of areas in which your performance could use some work?

In Chapter 1 we discussed the scope of practice for various roles. Review those again, keeping in mind your own particular set of skills and competencies. Can you honestly say that you have mastered the full role at this new level of education? This is different from comparing your performance with those graduates of the program who you have observed working alongside of you. Maybe they have not mastered the role either or are not employed in a position where the role can be played out. When you feel a stab wound in your self-concept, try to rationally analyze the circumstances. Try to think of the way you play the role of nurse as something outside of "you." Your role of nurse is only one part of the total "you"; think of it as a part that can be set aside, tinkered with, polished up, added to—all without changing the essence or totality of "you."

Was the source of the stab wound an attempt at shaping a part of your nurse role that could use a little redesigning? If so, that is easy to work on. It does not mean any kind of a change in the essence of "you." Your value as an individual and a human being is never in question. Nor, in a very real sense, is your value as a nurse in question. You have already established the fact that you are a good nurse. You have years of informal and formal evaluations to tell you that you have been performing your nursing role at least adequately, and quite probably excellently. The criticism that caused that stab wound was aimed at how you play the *ideal* nurse role, not the role you have played in the past. Consider the "stab wound trigger" as a prime source of information to you. It tells you how your school defines the "ideal nurse" and gives you some very specific information about how you should display the characteristics of the ideal nurse.

Stay very alert to all clues faculty members give about how they define the ideal nursing role in this setting. The faculty certainly will not hide this information from you; it will permeate their lectures, the readings they assign you, the clinical conferences, and every other educational experience planned for you. The problem with experienced students is that they tend to discount these signals from faculty *if* the ideal role is some distance from the nurse–students' understanding and capabilities. For example, if the faculty spend two hours lecturing on the importance of ferreting out the seven characteristics of every symptom discovered during a health assessment, you can be quite sure that they consider this an important part of ideal nursing care. Regardless of how you feel about the practical implementability of this (or even it's worth in the nursing care of patients), you would be smart to display your ability to do this well.

Usually the most anxiety-producing aspects of figuring out the ideal role are the nebulous areas. For instance, you may hear a great deal about "holistic" nursing care, and you deduce that this faculty highly prizes such care. But what does this *really* mean in terms of the tasks set before you as a nurse–student? Does it mean always including family members in planning care? Does it mean always thinking about psychosocial aspects while you perform biophysical tasks? In what ways will you have to change your usual methods of dealing with clients so that you are displaying behavior which shows that you know how to give "holistic" nursing care (as defined by this faculty)? There are no pat answers to these questions. You will have to ask questions and "try on" some behaviors before you know for sure what they are looking for. The signals are all there; it is up to you to learn how to interpret them.

Do not waste your precious time and energy while in school bemoaning the fact that the ideal nursing role is not implementable in any real-life nursing service organization. You can tussle with how to implement the ideal role in the real world *after* you graduate. Your task while in school is to sharply define the ideal nursing role, as it is taught in the school you are attending, and then to display as many characteristics of the ideal nurse as you possibly can when you are given opportunities to do so. Look upon the chance to play the "ideal nurse" as a privilege;

this is probably one of the rare times that circumstances and situations will let you do it. Why do educational institutions emphasize ideals and a future orientation? The faculty teach to an ideal nursing role because they believe that this is the best way to foster the highest-quality nursing care in the real world. They hope that you will become so comfortable, skilled, and committed to ideal nursing care that you will find ways to implement it in your work setting, now and in the future. They want you to raise your internal standards. These "internalized standards" become the day-to-day yardsticks for how people act in the real work setting: what decisions are made, what activities take priority over other activities when not everything can be done, what is viewed as so important that it cannot be glossed over. In very real terms, your internalized standards become a measure of what you, as a health professional, will tolerate as acceptable nursing care in your work setting. High-quality care will only come about (academicians and many others believe) if those who practice nursing adhere to internal standards that reflect the best that is known about nursing.

REALIZING THE VALUE OF UNDERSTANDING ACADEMIC VALUES

We believe it is helpful for educationally mobile nurses to do some careful thinking regarding values. Values are expressions of the things that we believe are important; values motivate our behavior. It is important that you understand the values of the typical institution of higher learning so that you will be able to predict more accurately how people who are part of this world will act and behave. The values that you have learned in the workplace will not be the same as those in academia.

What are some of the values of academia? The following list would probably be a typical answer to that question; this list is neither exhaustive nor true of all academic settings. It is presented as an illustration of what we mean when we talk of "values."

1. *Rationality is valued in institutions of higher education.* This means that knowledge gained through scientific reasoning based on logic, proper research methods, and accepted theories is prized.

An outcome of this value is that academicians tend to place high worth on ideas or ways of doing things that are found in "the literature." "The literature" is a term used to describe all the journals, books, research reports located in miniaturized data banks, and other sources of written information found in higher education institutions. Presumably the ideas and theories present in "the literature" got there because they were generated through rational means: research, observations, theory building, or empirical testing. The more knowledgeably you can quote the literature of your field, the more persuasive you will be in having your own ideas accepted. People socialized into the academic world look to "the literature" as the source of authoritative knowledge. Just finding something written down may not win an argument, however. Sources vary in their acceptability as part of "the literature" of a field. Citing references found in a library is usually powerfully persuasive; citing the procedure book from your workplace may be persuasive only in a few instances.

2.   *Academic traditions are important.* Academicians, normally governed so strongly by rationality, become much less rational when dealing with the traditions of academia itself. For example, there is a growing body of literature and research which suggests that adults would feel more comfortable and perhaps learn more if higher education institutions would let the adult student write highly individualized objectives for each course. These suggestions have not been adopted, especially in those academic areas such as the health-related sciences where there is a vast amount of knowledge available. The traditional pedagogical approach in which the faculty set the objectives for each course continues to prevail. Academicians who may be stunningly unconventional in their approach to the theory or mechanics of their particular field of study typically become quite conservative when it comes to changing the academic setting itself. Academia is like any subculture in this respect; the traditions of the group tend to damp the forces of change.

3.   *Communication, both oral and written, is valued.* The format for communication tends to be rather formally defined in both areas. Your success as a student may very well hinge on your ability to communicate well.

4.   *Broad and liberal viewpoints are usually valued.* In most academic settings, the less ethnocentric and provincial the student proves to be, the more successful the student role performance is. A world view that sees a broad picture, that is rich in complexity, is generally reinforced by the inhabitants of academia.

Some academicians may hold broad general viewpoints while they are simultaneously picky about little details. This is understandably confusing to students. Usually the pickiness arises from an attempt to hold students to "ideal" standards.

5.   *Adherence to high ideals is valued.* Because academia deals in

ideas, not products or services, there is less of a tendency to settle for expedient solutions to problems. Maintaining ideals is usually considered more important than meeting the needs of individuals.

6.   *Time is an important element in academia.* The credit awarded for attending classes is closely linked to the time spent in the classroom. Deadlines for producing papers or for taking tests or for performing some other academic task may be rigidly enforced; people may be punished for failing to comply with various time deadlines.

7.   *Searching for "truth" is a prime motivating factor in academia.* Institutions of higher education benefit society by producing and transmitting knowledge. Knowledge is generated and shared in academia. Today's "truth" may well be tomorrow's abandoned theory, however, as knowledge is generated and modified through additional study and discovery. Thus an attitude of objective inquiry and a willingness to change one's thinking in the face of rational evidence are usually prized in the academic world.

8.   *There are differences in the status, power, and ranking of people in academia.* There is both a bureaucratic hierarchy (which has service employees at the bottom and the president or chief administrative officer of the institution at the top) and a hierarchy of faculty members (which usually puts instructors at the bottom and full professors at the top). Students often wonder where they fit in this social system. Many times students feel they are at the absolute bottom of any hierarchical arrangement in academia. However, that is too simplistic an analysis, we believe. In some ways students can be very powerful: They may have important input into the evaluation of faculty members, which has a bearing on tenure decisions, for instance, and they can exert influence on the curriculum and governance of a school.

In addition to differences in the status of individuals, there is an informal ranking of academic disciplines and majors. On some campuses, nursing may be the largest program in terms of numbers of students enrolled. This may very well enhance the power and prestige of the nursing department. In other, usually larger institutions, nursing may have much lower relative status because the nursing unit does not do much original research, or get large federal grants, or have faculty members who hold prestigious and powerful offices within the university organization. The informal ranking of the nursing department within an institution probably follows the ranking of the profession of nursing in society as a whole: usually lower than medicine, but about equal to education and the social sciences.

9. *Growth and change are valued.* Most teachers define learning as a "change in behavior." They expect students to change, will reward change, and are disappointed when change in behavior does not occur. I once asked fifty people who came to me for advisement when entering a school of nursing if they expected to change as a result of participating in the nursing school. The new high school graduates in the sample clearly expected to change as a result of the educational experiences: They were going to become nurses. The experienced nurses (both L.P.N.s and R.N.s) in the sample, however, could foresee very little change ahead for themselves. They were going to stay the same, in spite of the educational experiences. They did not expect to change their nursing behavior, nor did they expect to change as individuals. It is easy to imagine the friction resulting from students who do not expect change coming under the direction of faculty members who define their tasks as producing change in students.

In fact, most of the values listed previously can be seen to conflict in some way with some of the values of the typical workplace. Workplaces are organized around productivity and efficiency. "Getting the job done reasonably well" is the overwhelming value in most places that employ nurses (or anyone else, for that matter). Adherence to the rules and procedures of an organization is seen as essential to the smooth functioning of complex health-care facilities. Perfection in performance is always tempered by the need for delivering adequate, safe, acceptable care to all clients. Maintaining the smooth-functioning status quo is preferable to any original and untried idea that could have a negative impact on productivity.

As a skilled nurse (and presumably thoroughly socialized into the values of the workplace) how do you become also a skilled citizen of academia? It is primarily a matter of *adding* new dimensions to your role performances so that you incorporate the values and skills prized in academia into your repertoire of behavior. In addition to being skilled at charting tersely and accurately, and utilizing an acceptable vocabulary, you learn to write twenty-page care plans that cover every aspect of a client's status. You will probably never be asked to write twenty-page care plans in your workplace, but you will have had the experience of having to think through every possible problem, intervention strategy, and evaluation measure presently known. This experience will help you to think more broadly when next you are faced with writing a succinct, usable care plan in your workplace. Your performance in your workplace has become more sophisticated, but it still is congruent with the values and roles of that institution.

COPING EFFECTIVELY
WITH STRESS

The cumulative amounts of stress from all sources—the RTSS role changes, the life-style changes, the growth and developments changes—can overwhelm an individual, even though that person is well aware of how these stresses arise and is equipped with the tools to deal with the stresses. The obvious strategy for dealing with very high stress levels is to attempt to reduce some or all of the sources of stress. It may mean cutting down on the number of roles one plays; it may mean cutting back one's involvement, perhaps temporarily, in certain roles. Here are some strategies we have seen nurses use successfully in reducing their stress levels:

1. Reduce the amount of time spent in the workplace to the absolute minimum needed to keep afloat financially.

2. Reduce the semester's course load to less than full time.

3. Resign from extraneous social clubs, with the promise, if you really enjoy them, to visit occasionally and rejoin later when you are out of school.

4. Negotiate workplace schedules with the employer so that blocks of time at work are longer, but less frequent. For instance, employers may permit twelve-hour shifts three times a week in lieu of five eight-hour shifts.

5. Implement some relaxation techniques that work.

6. Increase your aerobic physical activity: swimming, jogging, bicycling.

7. Establish interim goals that you know you can achieve. Celebrate these "mini" goals with friends and families. You will feel that you are making progress.

Other parts of this book explore stress-management techniques in more detail. The point we are trying to make here is that no matter how sophisticated you become in playing the student and ideal nurse roles, or how comforted you are by the knowledge that all nurses experience RTSS to some extent, you can still find school traumatic just because the totality of your life is filled with stress at this time. The only remedy for this is to reduce the sources of stress.

PUTTING IT ALL IN PERSPECTIVE

Returning to school is a major decision and change point in the lives of nurses who do it. Those who successfully complete school, both in terms of earning their degrees and in emerging from RTSS as bicultural ambassadors, come away from the process with bright futures: Their career paths now have many additional options, their personal competencies are enhanced, their understandings and viewpoints are broadened. They have grown, changed, and will forever be different as people and as nurses.

But what about those who were not as successful? How about those for whom the RTSS stresses were overwhelming? How about those who simply *did not change* as a result of returning to school? Is it the end of the world? Dropping out, failing out, or just sliding through school are neither sinful nor illegal. An unsuccessful school experience may have a minimal impact on one's career, especially if the nurse is content with the present position. There are many explanations for an unsuccessful school experience: perhaps the timing was wrong, maybe the mix of personalities was unfortunate, perhaps the necessary resources were just not available. Perhaps it takes time—as long as two or three years—to come to grips with the interpersonal tensions one experiences during school; before that time the nurse may be reacting so emotionally to the negative experiences that the positive aspects of the return to school are simply lost. An unsuccessful experience at one point in your life does not preclude a later successful experience.

RTSS is a process that can be viewed as a series of transitions that develop a new set of role performances in the individual, with resulting changes in the role performance of other members of the role set. Experiencing RTSS teaches a person about the *process* of going through transitions. Once you have gone through a set of role transitions, you know how you react under such circumstances. The next time you are confronted with the opportunity or necessity for making a series of role transitions you will know more about how that feels; you will have more insight into how you can deliberately manage these transitions and how you can influence their outcome.

Thus, even if your return to school was less than successful in terms of reaching the bicultural ambassador level, or of obtaining the educational credential you desired, or of developing a set of competencies you expected to master, there is an excellent chance that you have learned about role transition: You have a sense of how flexible you are about role changes, you know more about yourself and how you feel about role changes, you have tested the limits of your capacity for change, and you may have observed your own resiliency in the face of formidable obstacles. Such self-knowledge can only be invaluable. It will hold you in good stead for a life that will be filled (as most lives are) with numerous and sometimes wrenching role changes.

PART THREE
GROUP HELP AND SELF-HELP

9

Developing Formal and Informal Support Systems

Jan Thornburg, R.N., M.S.N.

By now you are familiar with the theory and process of the returning-to-school syndrome. Other chapters have described how educationally mobile nurses move from an initial honeymoon stage to a stage of disappointment, frustration and anger, and then on to conflict resolution. You may have already experienced some of the emotions that returning to school generates. You may think, "If only I can live through the next few years, I'll get back to my normal way of living."

But gritting your teeth and vowing that you will make this school experience work will only add more stress to your already stressful life. Furthermore, you will not be the same after you finish school; your life will not return to the normalcy that you remember before you entered school. School will change your perceptions and behaviors. These next school years are an opportunity for you to grow and to develop new ways of perceiving yourself, both personally and professionally. One way to move through this role transition is to develop support systems that will help you to resolve your troubled thoughts and feelings. This support can be either an informal or a formal support system; each has its benefits and possibilities for growth.

INFORMAL SUPPORT SYSTEMS

Family and Friends

Informal support systems are those that students in any field of study develop to help get through the stress of test taking, paper writing, library research, and adjusting to new instructors and ideas. One source

135

of support may come solely from your circle of family and friends. You may share anecdotes of clinical experiences and feelings of frustration and anger with them. They may comfort you with statements such as, "I know you can do it, just stay in there" or "It must be awful to have to take those challenge exams!" This kind of support feels good and is very necessary.

A family member or friend can give you support, but they may not be able to help you through the role transition of returning to school. They may be unsure of how to respond to your complaints about school. They may slowly pull away from you by changing the subject or by interrupting your complaining. This withdrawal may make you feel that you are, once again, alone in your turmoil.

Your family and friends can offer only a certain amount of support. They can neither validate your experiences nor challenge your perceptions. If they did challenge you or encourage you to move away from the complaining, you might feel betrayed. The roles of family members and friends do not include the expectation that they will act as change agents. Rather, they can support you and provide a sympathetic listening ear.

Other Students

Another source of informal support for returning nurses is other students. They are able to validate what you see and hear. They are experiencing their own role transition turmoil and can confirm what you are experiencing. This validation will help you to feel that you are not alone. You will also learn that you are not crazy, that your views and feelings are based in reality, and that you can trust your own perceptions. The students who use each other for support seldom miss a chance to meet together: in the hallway between classes, over coffee or drinks in the lounge, in car pools, or after clinical hours.

Returning nurses may initially have a difficult time seeking out others and spending time with them. You have developed family and social roles that structure your time; when faced with adding new people into your social system, you may decide that you do not have the time or energy to seek out other students. Despite this reluctance, if you find other peers and begin to share your perceptions, opinions, and feelings, you will begin to offer feedback that helps group members to achieve some resolution of the conflicts that returning to school generates.

Perhaps one of the most important aspects of informal support is learning new ways of coping in a safe, nonthreatening situation. While sitting around a cup of coffee, one nurse may relate how a clinical instructor structured the challenge exam. She shares feelings about the instructor's expectations. All those who listen are gathering valuable information on how to meet these role expectations. They may not like what they hear, some may voice strong opposition and feelings of resentment, but all have heard information on how to survive. And all that information is free for the taking. No one has to admit to being scared, anxious, or angry. No one has to risk asking questions that might expose inner turmoil. Instead, each is able to get information in a safe, covert manner.

An unfortunate result of this kind of support is that you may continue to silently judge your own merit and performance as you compare yourself with the one who is speaking. You may judge yourself as inadequate because you do not know the material as well as the speaker seems to know it. You may feel you are doing something wrong because you do not do what the speaker says. This silent, personal judging helps to perpetuate your low self-esteem, which further adds to your turmoil. You may also be less willing to risk exposure of feelings and thoughts that somehow do not meet the approval of all those in the group. Consequently, you do not share and so do not get feedback; thus you may continue to feel anxious and confused.

FORMAL SUPPORT GROUPS

Formal support groups pick up where informal groups stop. These more organized, goal-oriented groups prevent their members from silently judging themselves and from staying alone with their misperceptions and tumultuous feelings. The group goals require members to commit themselves to active participation. Members agree to share their thoughts and feelings, as well as to give and receive feedback from others. This feedback mechanism stimulates members to let go of their old ways and thoughts and to choose a new way from the many options that are generated in the group.

Formal groups have a leader who not only shares personal thoughts and feelings, but who also keeps the members focused on specific topics and helps them to communicate more effectively with each other. The leader is aware of the process of change and how to help members to use change concepts in their own lives.

Change Process in Groups

The change process is a succession of steps that leads to new patterns of thinking and behaving. The first step is discovering and clarifying what you want or need in your life. If you are similar to many educationally mobile nurses, this clarifying step may be difficult, because you have not spent a lot of your time defining your own needs. Instead, you are schooled and socialized to define the needs and wants of others. Your personal needs can range from clearly defining what you want from your educational experience to what you need from your family while you are taking on the new student role.

The next step is exploring with other group members how you can meet your needs. You can get ideas from others on the various ways you can survive in the educational system, how you can talk to faculty members, how you can better organize your time, and how you can ask your spouse for different support while you study. This exploration of new ways of behaving and thinking is an intellectual exercise that all recognize. What often happens after you have gathered all the new ideas is that you find yourself unable to make a choice of how you want to change and consequently stay with the old, unsatisfying ways of thinking and feeling. The group leader can identify that you are stuck and help you to move to the next step: discovering the emotionally laden feelings and perceptions that keep you from changing.

Emotions can stop you from changing. In fact, emotions can act to sabotage our best laid plans. Therefore, it is vital that you have a safe, supportive group that will help you to discover how you are stopping yourself from asserting your needs and from getting what you need. These resistances to change are based on old patterns and decisions that you made when you were younger. You may have learned, for example, that you can take care of others, both patients and family, but you cannot meet your own needs. Often we are so socialized into this role that we do not even know what we want or need; we may have made the decision that our needs do not count. This painful awareness, when explored in the group, can help you to know better how you might act in the future. This self-awareness can also help you to make the different personal decision that you do have needs and that it is all right to get them met. Most resistances to change carry a similar emotionally laden component. When they are expressed and explored, they lose their power to stop us from growing and changing.

The last step in the change process involves practicing behaviors and communicating in new ways. Meleis (1975) refers to this practicing as role supplementation that helps to clarify and use the new role behaviors. The group is a safe place to practice asking for support and for discovering words that best communicate to others.

How to Form a Group

By now you may be sold on the benefits of formally organized groups, but you do not know how to get started. The first step is to get together a group of R.N.s who are experiencing the same turmoil and conflict.

You may already know each other because of your informal contacts out of class. Or some of you may realize that there are others just like you who seem to be on the edge of the student classes, and not really a part of any gathering. All you need to do is begin asking if others feel the same way that you do and you will generate the interest for a group.

Next you need to find a leader, someone who knows about how groups function and who is aware of how to help people through role transitions. These people can be found on psychiatric nursing faculties, at student mental health centers, and in graduate programs for psychiatric nursing.

My experiences as a leader of R.N. groups began when I was a student in graduate school taking course work on group process. I realized that, as I talked to my peers at coffee breaks, they were experiencing feelings and thoughts similar to mine. I talked to a faculty member who agreed to supervise me as a leader, and soon the group was meeting once a week during the lunch break. I also have experience leading a group for R.N.s as part of the faculty in a B.S.N. program. The examples I use in the remaining part of the chapter are from these experiences and seem to express the major issues and feelings of R.N.s during this transition time.

Getting Started

Most group theorists agree that the beginning phase of group process is centered on getting to know one another, developing a common bond of communication, and developing the norms that govern the behavior of the group members. You will probably begin by sharing feelings of anger, resentment, frustration, and disappointment. The courses are not what you expected, the instructors fail to be the mentors that you envisioned, and clinical challenges are demeaning and belittling. You may share the added role complication of being a student on the same unit where you work as an R.N.

Difficulties with your family may be shared. Because of your school commitments, your spouse may be unhappy about the lack of time for you to be together. One group member, for example, shared that the only time she could study at home was at night when everyone went to bed. However, her husband was unhappy with this because she was not with him. Another student shared that she was frustrated because the only time she could study was from 5 A.M. until breakfast. Consequently, she was too tired in the evening to be with her family. Another student shared her guilty feelings when her four-year-old son complained that he did not have a "real mom" now that she had gone back to school.

Many times group members voice questions such as "Why do I want my BSN anyway? "How come I'm such a masochist to do this to myself?" "Don't the instructors trust us with anything?" "What good does it do to study these nursing theories? I've gotten along fine up until now without them!"

After two or three group meetings, you feel that someone at last understands and you are not alone in your misery. You also know that you aren't crazy or misperceiving the entire experience; others have gone through the same emotions and situations. We now have a group of griping, complaining nurses who no longer feel isolated and alone. Sound familiar? Does this scene bring back your experiences of groups of nurses on hospital units who spend time going over and over their complaints and never moving on to changing their behavior or altering their environment?

Formal support groups can stay at this level of group development. The members of these groups feel stuck. They leave the group session feeling negative and helpless. Some may feel more angry at those who have power, that is, the instructors and administrators. Some may feel more stress and anxiety from the rumors and talk of dread and woe that are shared. Most of the topics of conversation focus on events that happened in the past and outside the group or on people who are not present in the group. These symptoms of a stuck group can be detected by members who become dissatisfied with the process of the group and no longer feel supported but pulled down by the interactions.

It is important that formal support groups have a leader to prevent a negative, stuck group from developing. A leader will help you to move into the working stage where you begin to focus on your own beliefs and values, feelings and behaviors. A leader brings the focus of the group from events outside the group that cannot be changed to behaviors and feelings that each of you have in the group. This refocusing helps you to see that you are the one who can change and learn new role behaviors.

Working Stage: Theme of Powerlessness

The move from griping and complaining to working on changes occurs as group members begin to identify themes of powerlessness. When you express your anger at having to prove your skills to an instructor, you are responding to your loss of credibility and power. Similarly, when you describe the frustration of not having any spare time, you are responding to a perceived sense of powerlessness; as a student, you are not able to control and live your life as you once did.

The student role is often viewed as being powerless. You are not expected to challenge instructors regarding what they are teaching. You are expected to let go of evaluating yourself and to give that responsibility to instructors who have the power to fail you or to affect your grade-point average. You are expected to perform upon the instructors' requests and to respond to their time schedules for paper writing and test taking. You are expected to drop family, social, and work obligations and to devote your time to school.

All these role expectations are a part of the educational system to which you are expected to comply. In fact, the process of becoming a "good student" is similar to becoming a "good patient": don't rock the boat, don't question the system, and learn to survive by taking on the new role behaviors. As a nurse you may have a difficult time with these expectations and may view them in a negative way. This negative perception helps to perpetuate your poor self-esteem and heighten your sense of powerlessness and loss of identity as a credible, responsible person. However, being a student can also be perceived in a positive manner.

An Example   A group member changed her perception of a clinical challenge exam. She had a negative experience in the clinical area where she became increasingly disorganized, nervous, and tense as the challenge progressed. She made some errors and could not answer some easy questions that the instructor asked. She passed the exam but felt inadequate and dumb. She was worried that she would respond in a similar manner in the next challenge. As group members shared their responses to the exams, she felt less isolated and realized that others were experiencing similar feelings of tension and stress.

The group leader then focused on the upcoming challenges and how they could be handled differently by the R.N. students. After group discussion, the members decided that they needed to move from a position of defending their actions to one of initiating and creating their experiences, a move from passivity and powerlessness to activity and effectiveness. One member suggested that the challenge exam offered the opportunity for them to be only responsible for one or two patients instead of an entire unit. Being a student would allow them time to carry out comprehensive assessments and care. They would feel less rushed and less task oriented. They would not have to be responsible for all doctors' orders, every telephone call, and every question that needed answering regarding patient care. Instead, the scope of responsibility would be limited, a very positive and refreshing aspect of being a student. They would be free to initiate their pet projects to improve patient care.

Let go of being responsible? Is that really possible for nurses? All of us are responsible; being an R.N. is responsible, being a student who also has a family and continues to work is responsible. Super responsible! But being a student again gives you permission to let go of some of that responsibility, some that you do not need to assume. The student role allows you to be less responsible for others and more responsible for yourself. You can now be responsible for identifying what you can gain from every experience as a student. This means that you can actively seek out newness and actively consider how the theories or new skills fit for you. You can actively use others in your group to explore new ideas and behaviors instead of remaining powerless, disgruntled, and unhappy.

Theme of Total Immersion

Another theme that emerges in the support group is the reliance on the student role for every source of validation, identity, and self-esteem. Some educationally mobile nurses begin to place too much emphasis on making it as a student. They set aside many of the roles that have proved to be supportive and that provided them with identity and a sense of accomplishment. The student role becomes one of too few roles. They worry too much about making straight A's, or writing the perfect paper, or performing flawlessly in the clinical area. They value what the instructors say so much that they are emotionally crushed when they receive any negative feedback. Their perpective on how much importance should be placed on only one aspect of life is lost.

An Example   One student began to see that she was placing such emphasis on making good grades, reading the assignments, and writing papers that her family was feeling left out. All her roles (mother, wife, sister, cook, lover) had been put on the shelf. She no longer acted out her mother role with her children, but expected her husband to take over the mothering while she studied. She no longer spent time with her husband in the wife role because of her total student immersion. She felt guilty when members of her family would complain or attempt to bring her back into the roles she had set aside. The group helped her to see that she was relying too heavily on the student role as her sole means of identity and self-worth. She saw that she valued the grade on her paper more than time spent with her family. She learned that she gave her instructors power to judge her behavior completely and had lost perspective on her life. She needed to occupy several roles selectively in her life so that she could gain self-worth and a sense of identity.

Another theme, different from the total immersion in the student role, is feeling overwhelmed with the student role expectation. Returning R.N.s are mothers, wives, and nurses. These roles have many expectations and the student role is yet another set of behaviors. Those who feel overwhelmed with these added expectations need to learn how to assign priorities to roles and how to compartmentalize them.

An Example   One group member who felt overwhelmed described how she could not let go of worrying over tests and assignments while she was around her family. She would go through the actions of comforting her child over a broken toy while feeling guilty over not studying. She would think that she should be spending time with her family instead of reading. Consequently, she was never fully with her family nor fully concentrating on her studies.

She felt disorganized and overwhelmed with all the expectations and responsibilities, and she knew she was not effective in any one of the roles. The group helped her to think through how much time she needed to study, when was the best time for her to study, and where she did her best concentrating. She was able to make a contract with herself to spend two hours a day studying in the library in the morning. She then had evenings to spend with her family. She would work on not worrying about her school obligations because she had a specific plan for study. She was able to see that she could separate the different roles in her life and concentrate her energy and time as needed. She felt she had gained control over her life and was not so powerless.

Groups can help their members discover how to compartmentalize roles—to totally be in one situation with focused concentration. As nurses you have learned how to be fully with one patient at a time, to give full attention to that one person in spite of many other distractions. Or you fully concentrate your attention on transcribing doctors' orders while other activities swirl around you. As you talk to others in the group, you can share many examples of efficiently performing one task or one role at a time. This will result in fewer feelings of being overwhelmed or worrying over all that needs to be done.

The group can also develop a series of strategies for preparing for school assignments. Perhaps these strategies will involve affirming your own ability and experience in writing papers or realizing that you can trust yourself and you do not have to waste your energy worrying about this aspect of being a student. Perhaps it will mean planning specific times to research and prepare a paper. Perhaps other group members will decide to meet together to help each other study. This serves to concentrate the energies of the members and will do much to relieve feelings of anxiety and stress.

Internalizing New Professional Behaviors

Another theme that emerges in a support group is the learning of new professional behaviors that are a part of the nursing program. In the group you can practice behaviors that contribute to being an effective change agent, behaviors of negotiation and assertion. Both are similar to the process of change that has been outlined earlier in the chapter. All involve determining what you think and feel, clarifying what you need or want, and then following through with actions that will bring about the identified changes.

An Example   One group member described a scene with a doctor who was angry with her thorough report of a patient that included a detailed psychosocial history. The doctor interrupted her and insisted that she proceed to report the findings from her physical exam. The R.N. felt put down and invalidated by the doctor's interruption and also felt confusion over what her role expectations were in that particular setting. The group members helped her to express her feelings of anger and hurt at being invalidated. They supported her in her emotional responses and helped her to express them in the group. The next step was to determine what the student wanted to happen. What did she want from the doctor? After discussion, she was clear that she wanted to continue the psychosocial evaluations, that she valued their importance, and that she was acting as a professional nurse by fulfilling these role behaviors. She also wanted the doctor to listen to her and to understand the value that she placed on these assessment data. The clarity of what she wanted was a relief for her. She was not confused over her role and felt strength and assurance because of this clarity.

New Behaviors

But how do you follow through with your wants? How do you tell the doctor you want him to listen to you? How do you deal with your feelings of anxiety over the forthcoming confrontation and negotiation?

These "hows" of new professional behavior are some of the most valuable and helpful aspects of support groups for nurses. Answering these "how" questions after you are clear on what you are thinking and feeling is the exciting component that is absent from the informal support groups.

One way to learn how to assert your needs to other professionals is by role playing. Maybe you are saying, "Oh no, not more role playing. That's so silly, we did too much of that in school." You may have role played scenes in nursing school about how to talk with patients or how to use therapeutic communication skills. You may have felt uncomfortable and silly. However, in support groups, role playing has a different flavor. You are not working with strangers but have formed a cohesive group that has already shared intense, intimate feelings. There is a feeling of safety such that you feel free to risk trying new ideas and actions. The role-playing topics are extremely interesting because they affect you intensely; the role playing of topics that focus on acquiring new intellectual skills are usually less engaging.

An Example   The group member who described the doctor's reaction to her in-depth history taking was able to discover how intensely she felt when she role played the scene with another group member. She began to re-experience frustration, anger, and pain because of the physician's invalidating behavior. She expressed these feelings by being confused and then bursting into tears. (Does this sound familiar? Nurses becoming frustrated and angry, and then expressing it by crying? And then feeling angrier because the crying seems to make one feel smaller and even more humiliated?)

With the help of the group the student explored how to respond to the doctor by expressing her anger and hurt feelings without the humiliating tears. She then practiced asking the doctor for what she wanted from him.

Another student used role playing to learn how to respond to an instructor who seemed to be asking more from the student than the student thought was appropriate. In fact, role playing can be used for any situation in which learning new responses and new behaviors is a part of taking on a new role (Meleis, 1975).

Assertion or Compliance

So far we have discussed the change process and assertion concepts that will help you in role transitions. We have noted that becoming a "good student" is similar to becoming a "good patient." You need to go along with role expectations in order to survive. Both of these concepts, (1) asserting needs and wants and (2) complying with expectations, are necessary for each of us to survive in the academic world, as well as in all other aspects of our lives. But when do you assert yourself and when do you comply? How do you know which one to do in a certain situation?

The common components of both actions are knowing (1) *how*

you feel and (2) *what you want.* From this position of clarity you can decide the best course of action. This decision is made even easier when you are in a group that agrees on a course of action to follow. When you know clearly that you are angry because of an interaction with an instructor and you know specifically what you need from the particular situation, you can decide if it would be better to assert your needs and ask for changes or to comply because the instructor is not open to negotiations. If you decide *not* to assert your needs, you do not have to feel defeated or powerless. You can help each other to find ways to survive with the instructor, to let go of being defensive and to find out what you can learn in the situation. You may also collectively decide that numbers carry more weight than one single voice. Perhaps all of you will decide, as a group, to gather data and present a grievance or request in a formal, organized manner.

The major issue is that you are clearly making choices on how to act; this is an active, participating, alive position. The old way—feeling victimized, powerless, and angry—is a passive, isolating, static position that does not lead to feelings of self-worth. The group can help each individual identify the available options. There is no formula for knowing whether to comply or assert. There is no one right way for each individual. Instead, there is an ongoing process of knowing yourself, what you want, and choosing options that make the most sense for you.

SUMMARY

Nurses who return to school should seek avenues of support to help meet the role transition traumas that come with learning the student role and the new professional roles. The most readily available source of support is your peers. You can validate each others' feelings, experiences, and perceptions and help each other change behaviors and perceptions so that you can be an active participant in your education instead of being a defensive, resisting nonlearner.

In a group of formally organized students, you can readily share your feelings of frustration, confusion, and anger. You are not alone in these unhappy, uncomfortable feelings. You can begin to pool your ideas as to how to survive in the new educational environment. You can help each other to practice assertive behaviors that you will carry with you when you reenter the work world with your new degree. Most important is your increased awareness of yourself and your ability to clarify your thoughts and feelings in order to make choices from among the many options that are now open to you in every aspect of life.

REFERENCES

Meleis, A. "Role Insufficiency and Role Supplementation: A Conceptual Framework," *Nursing Research* (July–August 1975), p. 264.

Supplemental Readings

Glaser, J., and K. Horvath. "A Tool for Dealing with Nursing Problems," *Supervisor Nurse* (April 1979), pp. 46–52.

Grissum, M., and C. Spengler. *Womanpower and Health Care*. Boston: Little, Brown & Co., 1976.

Hinshaw, A. *Socialization and Resocialization of Nurses for Professional Nursing Practice*. NLN Publication 15-1659. New York: National League for Nursing, 1977.

Loomis, M. *Group Process for Nurses*. St. Louis: C. V. Mosby Company, 1979.

Malkemes, L. "Resocialization: A Model for Nurse Practitioner Preparation," *Nursing Outlook* (February 1974), pp. 90–94.

Randolph, B., and C. Ross-Valiere. "Consciousness Raising Groups," *American Journal of Nursing* (May 1979), pp. 922–924.

Sampson, E., and M. Morthas. *Group Process for Health Professions*. New York: John Wiley & Sons, Inc., 1977.

Yalom, I. *The Theory and Practice of Group Psychotherapy*, 2nd ed. New York: Basic Books, Inc., 1975.

10

Redefining Your Priorities While Managing Stress and Crisis

Shirley Curtis, R.N., M.S.

Autumn haze
rustling leaves
bustling students

line after line after line

how've ya been?
Good to see you again.

New clothes
Sharpened pencils
inky smell of open books.

A time to learn
make new friends
compete again

School daze.

DEFINING PRIORITIES ON YOUR OWN

Returning to school was much simpler when you were younger. It was the expected thing for you to do each fall. Family, friends, and society (even you) knew what you would be doing when September rolled around. You may or may not have liked the foreclosed decision that returning to school was an obligation of youth defined by law. But you complied; willingly or defiantly, you complied. Returning to school was a priority of your youth-time; a priority imposed and supported by others, not necessarily by you. You probably spent little time thinking about it.

This time it is different. Now that you are an adult, you are a dominant key member of the decision-making processes that affect you. There is another difference: you are returning to school with knowledge, skills, and experiences as a part of your personal repertoire of worldly coping abilities. You know you have abilities to offer your clients and others. You are not a dependent, compliance-bound child anymore.

Somehow, someway you have decided to become educationally mobile—to join the many nurses who are returning to school to earn a degree. What an important decision! It is one of those landmark choices that will have an impact on the rest of your life. That decision, as we know, was not mandated by law, your parents, or other imposing authorities; as an adult, you have chosen to add "returning to school" as one of your personal priorities. Your task is to fit this priority into the finite life you have remaining. Juggling this new priority with the other priorities you already have established in your life schema will require considerable attention from *you*—not your parents, not your boss. You!

Granted, you may have felt an external push to become educationally mobile. If you are very lucky you may have responded to a frequently reported "urge to go back to school." You may have the strong support of friends, spouse, or employer. Nevertheless, adding a new time-consuming priority to your already crowded life commitments is ultimately your responsibility. How do you go about successfully pulling off such an enormous task?

Before bounding (like a curious kitten) or tensing (like an experienced cat stalking new prey) into the college scene, it would be wise to sit down alone and think a bit. Ask yourself two very ordinary questions that can get very complicated in the answering:

How do I now spend the twenty-four hours of each day?

How important and significant are each of those activities *to me now*?

Notice the emphasis on the words *"to me"* and *"now"*. Start with a simple laundry list. Which of these do you have in your life?

A spouse or partner
Loving pets
A home to maintain

An automobile that requires periodic upkeep
Close friends
Elderly parents close by
Children needing varying degrees of your time and attention
Work commitments
Volunteer activities
A television that you watch
Regular magazine subscriptions
A busy telephone
Entertaining obligations
New books to read
A garden to tend
A bridge or golf group to meet
Shopping and other errands to run
Exercising (jogging, running, walking) to do each day

Yes. Yes. Yes. Obviously you are just like the rest of us. You have made a lifetime of conscious and unconscious choices as to how you spend your limited time. Now it is time to reassess the relative importance of each "time-spent" variable in relation to your new goal, educational mobility. Each of the dimensions of your life take time, precious time. You will need to start making time your slave, serving *your* purposes, rather than letting time become an anchor hanging heavy about you.

As you finish this laundry list of current time expenditures, you will probably find that some related thoughts have been blipping through your mind: "I certainly don't want *that* relationship to be damaged by my going back to school." Or "Gosh, I couldn't survive without my garden."

These thoughts are important; let them flow and expand until you can categorize each of your existing commitments into one of four categories. Category 1 should contain those priorities of your life that you do not want to relinquish under any circumstance. In fact, you might want them to become even more significant than they now are. Category 2 should include those activities you do not want to see vanish from your life-style but that are not as critical as those in category 1. Category 3 is time fillers that you really are not as interested in as you once were. You would like to reassess their relative importance to your sense of well-being. Some examples might be monthly potluck dinners with friends and their families, volunteer committee membership, Sunday lunch with your mother-in-law, your flower garden, or spring and fall housecleaning. Category 4 is those time consumers you would prefer to give up right now if only you knew how. The laundry, grocery shopping, lawn upkeep, household errands, bridge club, den mother, children's chauffeuring, or Friday afternoon happy hours might fall in this category. Anything that does not fit into one of these four categories should simply not be included in your list; you do not have the time to waste on them anymore. Get rid of them!

Now set up a paper pencil pyramid of your four categories of time commitments. Remember, these are your personal priority choices. Do it like this:

$$1^A \quad 1^B \quad 1^C \quad 1^D$$

$$2^A \quad 2^B \quad 2^C \quad 2^D \quad 2^E$$

$$3^A \quad 3^B \quad 3^C \quad 3^D \quad 3^E \quad 3^F$$

$$4^A \quad 4^B \quad 4^C \quad 4^D \quad 4^E \quad 4^F \quad 4^G$$

The initial configuration is not as important as your revised one. Reflect on the initial configuration and redo it the next day after giving each of those commitments serious thought. Then, without further thought draw a line through all of category 4. These time consumers may actually be that simple to give up. They can be zapped away with the line of a pencil! These time wasters have been successfully cast off by others; all you need do is learn to adapt their techniques for ignoring, buying, or negotiating away these time wasters' existence.

Many 3's can be treated in the same manner as the 4's. It is the 2's and especially the 1's that are tricky; they may cause you the most difficulty as you experience the returning-to-school syndrome (RTSS). Let's assume that you can problem solve the 4's and 3's on your own with your existing personal resources. In this chapter, we will move right along to the major problems, the 1's and 2's. An example will serve us best:

1^A	1^B	1^C	1^D
Spouse	Children	School	Work

2^A	2^B	2^C
Extended family	Close friends	Recreation

These are examples of top priorities for some people. Expect them to shift in relative importance from day to day and hour to hour. Anticipate the unexpected, be flexible, set limits when needed, "flow with the river" whenever possible. Above all else, be true to your *essential* self, which is partially defined by your personal priorities.

Do not be deceived. It will be impossible for you to meet all the expectations your important 1's and 2's would like to believe you can provide while you are adding the responsibilities of a student. Our desires and fantasies far outreach the realities of our energy and time. This is a fact. It is a fact that needs to be faced openly and without guilt. Far too long, America's upwardly mobile women have tried to live up to an unreal image of "Ms. Perfect." For you to achieve your educational goal, the people residing in your categories 1 and 2 must come to the understanding that they will need to give up some of their hold on you.

In dealing with your 1's and 2's, you will need your best negotiating skills. Start these negotiations *before* you start classes. Your own mind-set is crucial to your success in getting others to assume responsibilities you will not be able to continue as a student, so review your motivations. Do you *really* want, or need, to become upwardly mobile in your career? If so, you will need cooperation and assistance from others if they are to remain a part of your commitment pyramid. It is best for you to speak with conviction and to communicate very clearly what you need from others. If you do not think you can do this, get some advice and brush-up practice on your assertiveness skills.

The people you will have to be prepared to deal with repeatedly are those who will endeavor to make you feel guilty for wanting to improve your career capabilities. Perhaps it is a friend, an in-law, your mother, or perhaps your husband (heaven help you if it's all four). Your contribution to the dialogue will sound something like this: "I now have the opportunity to go back to school to get my degree. I'm excited about it and want to do it very much. It will be a lot easier for me if I have your support and help. You can help me by *doing the laundry—or accepting a postcard every two weeks instead of my usual weekly letter— or by being available to take care of Jamie if she should get sick during exam week.*"

Know what you want, what you need and be assured that you deserve (you do!) your day in the sun. Anticipate that, regardless of how well you plan and negotiate tradeoffs, a "fly-in-the-ointment" will inevitably appear. It may be a flat tire, a stopped-up sink, changes in child-care arrangements, or a late husband. You could choose to perceive these as major disruptions that affect you for days. Or you can make well-established contingency plans, which include a sense of "this is life" when these plans backfire.

If your 1's and 2's cannot accept the fact that returning to school is as important to you as some of their time commitments, then you may be in for some deep soul searching. Are they really concerned about you as an individual person? Are you serving merely as an extension of themselves or to make their life more gratifying? Best get some help if this becomes a big issue. Help is mandatory for those who find themselves involved with abusive (physical, verbal, or mental) "support" systems. You may find that if others cannot allow you the space, freedom, and support for growth then you can no longer afford to expend your finite lifetime in supporting their one-sided existence.

In addition to being able to define and negotiate with significant others your personal time priorities, you should master two additional interpersonal skills that will serve you well, especially while you experience the RTSS: (1) managing stress and (2) do-it-yourself crisis intervention.

STRESS MANAGEMENT

Stress management is best accomplished by *preventing* excessive stress. As a developing human being, you have already learned ways to deal with excessive stress. Perhaps you are the type of person who likes to sit down alone at the end of a hectic day to think through rough spots. Maybe you prefer to talk out your difficulties with a friend. Or do you storm about the house slamming cupboards doors and rattling pots and pans? Perhaps you latch onto the first person you see and proceed to get into a silly argument over trivia.

Students develop creative ways of dealing with the stress of returning to school. For instance, some students car-pooled to school and traded off driving so each could spend time silently withdrawing from conversation or meditating. Another student chose to allow herself permission to take short naps any time of the day or night depending on her schedule and her need to withdraw from too much stimuli.

Excessive stress for many returning-to-school students revolves around these issues: decreased income, a loss of role and status as a member of the health-care team (for those who quit work or reduce their hours), isolation from old friends due to the added commitment of class and study time, and the expectations of instructors that each nurse will develop and use new ways of perceiving and thinking about nursing. Many experienced nurses begin to feel powerless as their previous knowledge and skills are debated in class and challenged by predictions of what will be useful in future health care. In effect, you may experience a loss of authority status. That is not a pleasant feeling for anyone!

One way of coping with the loss of authority and status in the work setting is to immediately establish an authority and status position in the new role (student) and setting (school). For example, buy a college tee-shirt that, in a nonverbal yet graphic way, proclaims to the world "I'm a student and proud of it!" (It doesn't matter that you are forty-five years old—do it anyway!) Or become the class expert on how to use the library with all its marvelous but mysterious new technological devices. Many returning nurses like to become mentors for the new registrants each term. It can be fun teaching someone else how to by-pass the snags of registration, or how to procure used books, use student services, or just find their way around campus. Experienced and inexperienced nurses can make an exceptionally compatible support system.

One underlying principle you need to *always* keep foremost in your mind is this: stress in and of itself is not "bad." In fact, a relative degree of stress is good, even essential to success. There is a fine line between too much stress and an optimal amount of stress. That fine line is relative and individual. You need to learn to recognize your optimal stress load and strive to maintain it; it will keep you goal oriented. Your optimal stress load will be like a thermometer for you; it will signal the time to put on more self-discipline and pressure, as well as when to call into play your skills of crisis intervention.

At least three key indicators show that you are not pushing yourself hard enough: (1) your time management is out of control (papers are late or you are not prepared for class twice in a row); (2) your communications with category 1 people get garbled, and disquieting conflicts start to impede your best-laid plans; or (3) you experience too frequently the sensation "this isn't as bad as I thought."

When you decided to become educationally mobile, you chose both a rewarding and a demanding goal. If you fail to press yourself to "keep on top" of your category 1 priorities, you will soon find your personal stressors pushing the stress thermometer above normal. Different people experience different signs and symptoms of stress overload. Learn to recognize your own. Common ones are the following:

Facial tics

Speeding tickets, even accidents

Increased difficulty with weight control (this can go either way, too thin or too fat)

Becoming a "nit-picker" instead of finding the humor in human frailties

Abuse of alcohol or other drugs

"Fizzled out" sexuality

Distrust of your own capabilities

Too much time spent in rumination over the day's events

Disturbances in usual sleep patterns

These or other signs and symptoms of a stress overload should signal a red alert and immediately command your serious attention. Somehow your life is getting out of hand. Your deliberate, willful self needs to get it back in line with where your wise and calculating self wants to be five years from now.

As a nurse, you know that the major resource a client has for dealing with stress is his own personal strengths. Try using the nursing process on yourself as you seek ways to manage your own stress level. After you have pinpointed your signs of stress, assess your built-in strengths and resources. Is your:

sleep pattern adequate?

nutritional balance good?

pacing and alternation of mental and physical activities with self and others (study, work, and play) optimal?

level of commitment to your personal priorities clear to yourself and others?

biological cycle normal and regular?

sense of humor intact?

Gaining control of your life means making effective use of your existing support systems and other self-defined stress-reduction mechanisms. Some very effective stress-reduction techniques include meditation, jogging, time alone, prayer, and happy social times with old and new friends. Plan specific action steps you will take to make best use of your particular, unique strengths.

If your stress-overload indicators are "flashing red," you need to develop a detailed plan for reducing your overall stress load. Your plan should be implementable immediately. Take the action steps you have outlined and then evaluate the outcomes. Has your stress level been reduced? Are the "flashing red" stress-overload signals quieted down? Yes? Great! You have successfully managed stress. This is a skill that you will be able to use many times in your lifetime.

CRISIS INTERVENTION

Most students experience some anxiety, frustration, or perhaps a slight sense of disorientation when they initially set foot on campus. As they begin to get a feel for what it is like to be a student again, those emotions frequently give way to an excitement and a buoyant sense of lightness. The joy of doing something positive for yourself, for your future career expansion, and just being with others who enjoy learning adds incrementally to your new-found pleasure. This honeymoon stage of returning to school is similar to other experiences when one finds new adventures and temporarily forgets the old grievances in previous life roles. The degree of the emotional high will vary from student to student, and so will the dipping into lows that almost universally occurs to the returning-to-school adult learner. The deepest low for many educationally mobile nurses occurs when they encounter their first clinical nursing course. Generalized explanations of this phenomenon are varied; only you can explain your own, and it is very important to your future well-being that you do so.

It is painful to acknowledge that one is not free from the vulnerabilities that affect clients, classmates, professors, indeed, all humans. A disturbing sense of loss is common to all who dare to acknowledge their awakening awareness of inadequacy in a new role.

Many of us have not been taught, nor had the experience of sharing with a role model the nuances of how to survive (stronger than before) the mild depressions that precede self-acceptance. It is hoped that this brief discussion of crisis intervention for students submerging into RTSS will help you to learn how to cope successfully with the ubiquitous human experience of personal crisis. Having gained this self-knowledge, you will have a richer repertoire of life responses to lend to others for the remainder of your professional career.

Crisis can be defined as a level of stress beyond one's coping abilities. Returning to school can precipitate either situational or developmental crises. Few nurses returning to school actually experience stress beyond their coping abilities, but you should be aware that it can happen. Crisis-precipitating events and the responses to these events vary from individual to individual.

The first sign of a personal crisis that you should be alert for is the *sudden* loss of ability to cope with a life situation. That inability may be related directly to school or it may be intimately involved with one of your other category 1 or 2 self-defined priorities. Work–school schedule conflicts, arguments with spouse or partner, drinking while on duty, sexual acting out, or something as bland as a perceived inability to get an A in a nonnursing course could signal a crisis. It does not matter whether the impossible-to-deal-with situation is social, personal, or school related; it is just a common life occurrence that you cannot deal with right now.

How do you pinpoint the particular stressor that has your system overloaded to the point of malfunction? Look to the past twenty-four hours first of all. What was different about it? Was there a disagreement? An outright argument? Perhaps a perceived put-down? An ominous letter from a creditor? A child out of control? A flight from it all by spending an evening with a friend instead of studying? A family need you were unable to respond to? Search and introspect with honesty and persistence. You need to get a clear perception of the precipitating event before further problem solving can be done.

If you cannot locate a disrupting factor that occurred within the past twenty-four hours, go back through your memory of the past one to two weeks. Most situational crises have their origins in the recent past. Think of a time line that looks like the following:

Time Preceding Crisis	Past 1–2 Weeks to Past 24 Hours	I N T E R V E N T I O N	3–6 Weeks Later	
Life essentially OK	Things not OK		Things getting better	Life essentially OK
	Withdrawal from others			
	Tears, anger, dysfunction			
	Guilt, sleeplessness			
	Precipitating crisis event occurred in this time span			

You need to find "the" event, be it real, imagined, or distorted (that does not matter for now). Become a skilled detective with your inner-self; keep searching for the trigger that sent your priorities askew and your stress-management plan right out the window. Keep your mind on the task of defining the precipitating event. Don't glide over it!

You found "it"? Good! Now you are ready to get yourself back on track. It may not necessarily be pleasant, but the road to regrouping your self-esteem can now be plotted. Your goal is to get yourself *functioning* at your previous level. No one ever promised us that life would be easy. Our hope for future effectiveness and joy lies within our ability to use reliable support systems to get our wobbly self picked up out of the dust and trekking down the road again.

A common human error is to believe that adults should not need kind, nurturing understanding from other adults. Another myth is that children should be totally shielded from parental disequilibria. Children know and sense parental distress despite efforts to "carry on as usual." Why not openly share that you are having a particularly hard time? Simultaneously, reach out to old and new support groups for a fuller comprehension of your particular difficulty. Children are reassured (as are family and peers) when they know you have the ego strength to reach out for temporary help. Does it surprise you that seeking others' perspectives on your difficulties is viewed as a sign of strength? If so, perhaps it is because you have been exposed to too many overly dependent people who never learned how to reactivate their own coping abilities.

To safeguard yourself from becoming one of these forever dependent souls, it is necessary for you to continue working on your personal crisis beyond the identification and "reaching out to others" stages. Actively recall previous crises of a similar nature, either in your own life or someone else's. How was that crisis resolved? Did you take control of your own life by reorganizing your daily, weekly, or monthly schedule? Did you set up a home study center, which served as a constant reminder to you and others that "regular study time is necessary"? In essence, what you do when reactivating your coping abilities is to (1) reaffirm your commitment to your goal, (2) remember old techniques that helped you attain a similar goal in the past, (3) try some new mechanisms that you have seen respected others use, and then (4) stick to your plans, equipped with your own and others' borrowed techniques. Remain *active* in your thinking. Search for every known mechanism that promoted restoration to an optimal functioning of either yourself or another. Activity is the key to your resolution. Be active in talk with others. Be active in powerful self-talk in which you delete self put-downs and promote conscious reminders of your past successes. No more relying on nonverbal and indirect communication of your feelings and needs! It is too difficult and time consuming for others to recognize or understand the meaning of your passive communications. How can they help you when you need it most if you resort to obscure messages? If you have not learned before, *now* is the time to be honest and direct with yourself and trusted others. No pussy-footing! Choose your confidants well, muster your past coping skills (for example, changing your pace, writing letters or poetry, going to church, taking daily walks, phoning a friend you have not talked to in months, baking cookies "just like you used to," whatever it is simply *do it* whether you feel like it or not). Don't bottle up those "silly" tears! Encourage them, urge them all to come out! They will clear your lacrimal ducts!

Tears are still viewed by many as a sign of female weakness. But we also know they are a valid indicator of pain, which is the wellspring of compassion. Today many people are beginning to realize that the repetitive display of tears indicates that they have not yet had the opportunity to learn how to verbally express the frustration and hurt that underlies the tears. Others view crying as a manipulative behavior. With these various understandings of what tears mean, you need to allow yourself the opportunity to learn what they mean for you. Now is a "safe" time to learn this important lesson. Actively reaching out for and accepting help during a time of crisis is an intelligent strategy. Consider using the college counseling center; it is staffed by experts in crisis intervention who deal everyday with other students. Why not you?

The 1980s will be "the decade" of the nontraditional learner. Ask the college counseling center or your nursing advisor to help you establish a small group where you can meet with others who are experiencing similar stresses. With others like yourself you can teach and learn how to survive while continuing to achieve your important personal goals.

As your ability to read your stress-management thermometer becomes more keen, you will learn to intervene for yourself a degree earlier the next time. This means that your stress level will not progress to the crisis stage. Stresses, and sometimes crises, come to everyone. Be prepared to help not only your clients and yourself, but all those who help you to progress toward your ultimate goal.

One last note for those students who find, despite their best efforts at crisis intervention, that they simply must postpone their educational goals on a temporary basis. Every class seems to have at least one "drop out." Some students indeed must withdraw for a term or two for such reasons as illness of spouse, child, or self; having a baby; need to work full time to earn money to support the education desired; need for time to adjust to a family crisis such as a death or divorce; recovery from an automobile accident; overwhelming time commitments to elderly parents; and the like.

Faculty and students alike need to openly acknowledge the temporary withdrawal as a necessary coping strategy. To succumb to fear that such a withdrawal constitutes an absolute discontinuance of educational mobility is an irrational response to a common occurrence. Students who find themselves in this circumstance would do well to keep in contact with their educational colleagues and faculty advisors. An occasional coffee break back on campus can bridge the need for reassurance that the educational process will be reactivated at a future time. Biculturalism can still be achieved by able nurses despite unfortunate setbacks. As an upwardly mobile nurse, you will become biculturally wise and pluralistically accepting of yourself and others.

PART FOUR

UNDERSTANDING YOURSELF
AS STUDENT

11

You as an Adult Learner

Mary Jane Ferrell, R.N., M.S.N.

Have you ever heard the old line, "You cannot teach an old dog new tricks?" You may have fears, as you once again enter a nursing education program, that you are perhaps too old to learn. The belief that adults are too old to learn is certainly a myth, but it concerns many nurses as they return to formal educational settings.

In this chapter we will discuss adult learners. Even though generalities will be made, it is important for you to realize that you are a unique individual. You have your own interests, drives, motivations, expectations, and aspirations. You possess experiences, values, needs, goals, and ideas that cause you to behave differently from your colleagues. Your mental abilities, height, weight, in fact all your psychological, physiological, and anatomical measurements are unlike any other person's.

Therefore, you, as an adult learner, have qualities that are unique. However, you also share common concerns and similarities with others. It is these commonalities and the concerns that you may have about learning that we will explore in this chapter.

WHY ADULTS LEARN

You are one of the thousands of adults in the United States who is engaged in learning activities. Tough (1979) found, in defining the learning project as "a major, highly deliberate effort to gain certain knowledge and skill," that approximately 98 percent of the adults in his research sample were engaged in learning. Adults participate in various types of learning: organized learning activities, self-directed learning, and courses that award academic credit. Cross (1981, p. 79) states that this adult learning force can be pictured as a pyramid of learners. She explains,

> Its broad base consists of self-directed learners, a category that includes just about everyone. A smaller group, estimated at one-third or more of the population, participate in some form of organized instruction each year, and the tip of the pyramid consists of that very small proportion of adult learners who pursue college credit in a wide variety of traditional and nontraditional programs.

Why do adults such as yourself participate in learning activities (credit or noncredit)? Pioneer work in answering this question was reported by Houle in 1961. He studied a small group of twenty-two people who were identified as "continuing learners." Three subgroups emerged, but Houle pointed out that "these are not pure types; the best way to represent them pictorially would be by three circles which overlap at their edges. But the central emphasis of each subgroup is clearly discernible" (Houle, 1961, p. 16). The three types are as follows:

1. *Goal-oriented learners* who use education to accomplish specific objectives. "The continuing education of the goal-oriented is in episodes, each of which begins with the realization of a need of the identification of an interest . . . . The need or interest appears and they satisfy it by taking a course, or joining a group, or reading a book, or going on a trip" (Houle, 1961, p. 18).

2. *Activity-oriented learners* who participate primarily for the sake of the activity itself and not to learn subject matter or develop a skill. "[They] were course-takers and group-joiners. They might stay within a single institution or they might go to a number of different places, but it was social contact that they sought and their selection of any activity was essentially based on the amount and kind of human relationships it would yield" (Houle, 1961, pp. 23–24).

3. *Learning-oriented learners* who seek knowledge for its own sake. "[They] are avid readers and have been since children; they join groups and classes and organizations for educational reasons; they select the serious programs on television and radio . . . . [They] choose jobs and make other decisions in life in terms of the potential for growth which they offer" (Houle, 1961, pp. 24–25).

Tough found in his study various reasons why adults undertake learning projects. Several of these reasons related to knowledge and skill: intention of using the knowledge and skill, imparting it to others, or for future understanding or learning. In some projects, a large part of the motivation came from the expectation of receiving credit for learning. But regardless of their motivation, the adults experienced pleasure, self-esteem, and confidence. These feelings resulted from satisfying a curiosity or puzzlement, from the content itself, from practicing the skill, from learning successfully, from completing unfinished learning, or from enjoying the activity of learning itself (Tough, 1979, pp. 50–61). These reasons for undertaking learning projects look similar to Houle's classification of learners.

What type of learner do you tend to be? Are you goal oriented, activity oriented, or learning oriented? Remember, there are no pure types. Why are you continuing your nursing education?

ASSUMPTIONS ABOUT LEARNING

Adults Can Learn

One of the questions raised in the beginning of this chapter related to "am I too old to learn?" The answer is, "No, you are not too old to learn. Adults can learn effectively!"

In 1927 Thorndike reported for the first time his findings that the ability to learn declined only very slowly and very slightly after age 20. Later studies indicated that what actually declined was the speed of learning, not intellectual power, and that even this decline was probably minimized by continued use of the intellect (Knowles, 1970, pp. 49–50). There is physiological aging of cells that affects the sensory functions of vision, hearing, and reaction time. Therefore, because older people may not be able to see or hear as well or move as fast, they may feel they cannot learn.

Intelligence is usually measured by IQ tests, but there are controversies over the appropriateness of these conventional intelligence tests as measures of adult learning capacity. Questions also arise about the differences in results from cross-sectional versus longitudinal studies. However, there is a general conclusion that "normal, healthy adults can expect to be efficient and effective lifelong learners well into old age" (Cross, 1981, p. 161).

Adult learners whom Houle studied provided a wealth of support for the belief that adults can learn. Here is what five of the adults had to say:

> I had stopped formal studying for a period of fifteen years and upon resumption was quite surprised that the habit of learning was so easy to resume.

Instead of finding special problems, I found it less difficult—whether this represented a maturity on my part, or settled habits, or better powers of concentration, I could not evaluate.

I find learning easier as an adult because I have a more intense desire to acquire new knowledge and explore ideas. Understanding comes easier.

Learning comes easier today because the years have taught me to analyze problems better and come up with better solutions.

After twenty years, I found learning easier. I concentrated better, was more interested—consequently I learned more.

I felt more mature and in a better position to cope with what I wanted to learn. (Houle, 1964, pp. 20–21)

Therefore, the basic ability to learn remains essentially unimpaired during a person's life span, and if adults do not actually perform as well in learning situations as they could, the cause may be sought in the following factors (Knowles, 1970, p. 50):

Adults who have been away from systematic education for some time may underestimate their ability to learn, and this lack of confidence may prevent them from applying themselves wholly.

Methods of teaching have changed since most adults were in school, so that most of them have to go through a period of adjustment to strange new conditions.

Various physiological changes occur in the process of aging, such as decline in visual acuity, reduction in speed or reaction, and lowering of energy levels, which operate as barriers to learning unless compensated for by such devices as louder sound, larger printing, and slower pace.

Adults respond less readily to external sanctions for learning (such as grades) than to internal motivation.

You can learn. Perhaps one of the reasons why you continue to learn well is that you concentrate your learning in the area of experience in which your interests also lie. Thus your "motivation is substantial and, as everyone knows, wanting to learn is the greatest aid to learning. Adults of all ages can learn effectively and 'age has no veto power over learning'" (Kidd, 1973, p. 91).

Learning Is an Internal Process

Learning is an internal process that is controlled by you, the learner; it involves your whole being, your intellectual, physiological, and emotional functions. Knowles (1970, pp. 50–51) explains:

Learning is described psychologically as a process of need-meeting and goal-striving by the learner. This is to say that an individual is motivated to engage in learning to the extent that he feels a need to learn and perceives a personal goal that learning will help to achieve; and he will invest his energy in making use of available resources to the extent that he perceives them as being relevant to his needs and goals.

The central dynamic of the learning process is thus perceived to be the experience of the learning, experience being defined as the interaction between an individual and his environment.

THEORIES ABOUT LEARNING

There are many theories about learning that have been based predominately on studies of animals and children. One classification divides learning theories into the categories of behaviorism, cognitivism, and humanism.

Behaviorism

Behaviorists, such as Thorndike and Skinner, concern themselves with the observables of behavior, that is stimuli (S) and responses (R). "Strict behavioristic doctrine avoids any speculation about what is going on in the mind" (Dubin and Okun, 1973, p. 4). Therefore, this theory considers people to be passive; they are governed by stimuli supplied by the external environment. People can be manipulated, that is, their behavior can be controlled through proper control of environmental stimuli (Milhollan and Forisha, 1972, p. 13). The behaviorists point out that in the early stages of training (that is, during the acquisition of knowledge) it is very important to immediately reinforce the desired response. This type of reward assures learning and repetition of the desired behavior.

Programmed instruction, computer-assisted instruction, and other types of self-instructional methods are actually direct applications of theories formulated by behaviorists. These learning materials usually have the following characteristics (Srinivasan, 1977, p. 12):

1. Objectives must be clearly stated in specific and measurable statements that precisely describe how the learner will perform or "behave."
2. The learning tasks must be analytically designed in relation to the desired end behaviors.
3. Content must be broken into small steps that are easy to master.
4. The materials should provide a means for immediate feedback so that the learner will know if his response was correct.
5. The subject matter and activities must adhere to a prescribed sequence and process conducive to mastery.

6. The successful completion of each step and the chain of steps must provide its own reward or incentive.

7. The responsibility for ensuring that learning takes place must rest with the materials themselves as learning instruments and not with any instructor, leader, or helper.

Cognitivism

Whereas behaviorists see learning as a process by which behavior is changed or controlled, the cognitive theorists such as Bruner define learning in terms of growth and development of competencies (Knowles, 1978, pp. 7-8). They consider the cognitive structure of the individual to be of paramount importance for learning (Dubin and Okun, 1973, p. 4). Bruner's theory about the act of learning involves three almost simultaneous processes: (1) acquisition of new information, (2) transformation, or the process of manipulating knowledge to make it fit new tasks, and (3) evaluation, or checking whether the way we have manipulated information is adequate to the task (Knowles, 1978, pp. 25-26).

Bruner advocates the discovery approach to learning. Learners are not presented with the subject matter in its final form; they must organize the subject matter themselves (Dubin and Okun, 1973, p. 8). The learners are active in deciding what to learn, are not told what the instructor already knows, explore alternative solutions, and develop working strategies for handling new information. Therefore, the learners are actively involved in the knowledge-acquiring process, with the instructor cooperating in this discovery of knowledge.

Another theorist generally classified as a cognitivist is Piaget. He hypothesized that intellectual development proceeds through a sequence of stages, or levels of cognition. These are as follows (Wadsworth, 1979, pp. 40-41).

1. Sensory-motor stage (0 to 2 years): development proceeds from reflex activity to sensory-motor solutions to problems.

2. Preoperational stage (2 to 7 years): development proceeds to prelogical thought and solution to problems; consists of establishing relationships between experience and action.

3. Concrete operation (7 to 11 years): development proceeds to logical solutions to concrete problems.

4. Formal operations (11 to 15 years): development proceeds to logical solutions to all classes of problems.

Piaget states that prior to thinking about abstract ideas, an individual must undergo a period of physical manipulation of objects, using the basic principles upon which the abstraction to be developed depends (concrete operation). Until students have had many such manipulative experiences, they cannot generalize those concepts and become capable of abstract thought, the formal operational stage (McKinnon and Renner, 1971, p. 1048).

Piaget found that most Swiss children should be capable of abstract logical thought by age 15. Therefore, it was once assumed that all adults would achieve the formal level of thinking. However, McKinnon and Renner found that American college freshmen had not become formal operational (McKinnon and Renner, 1971, p. 1049). It is possible that many nurses who return to school may be concrete rather than formal thinkers. This is probably due to the somewhat rigid authoritarian style of learning used in many schools of nursing. Hence they may have difficulty understanding the abstractions of nursing theory that are presented in more advanced nursing education programs (Muzio and Ohashi, 1979, p. 530).

Humanism

The third type of learning theory is the humanistic viewpoint of learning, expounded by such persons as Maslow and Rogers. Humanists have in common their belief that each individual perceives the world in a unique (phenomenal) way, and only the individual can fully "know" this perceived world (Dubin and Okum, 1973, p. 9).

Maslow sees the goal of learning to be self-actualization, "the full use of talents, capacities, potentialities, etc. . . . developing to the full stature of which they [people] are capable" (Maslow, 1970, 150). Self-actualization is the fullest achievement of adult development. Characteristics Maslow associates with self-actualization are liking to do things well, the enjoyment of responsibility, interest in solving problems, preferring to work toward causes of one's own choice, refining and/or improving methods, and setting things straight (Maslow, 1971, p. 309).

Rogers, who takes his basis of learning from psychology, states that people act purposively, with the basic tendency being to actualize, maintain, and enhance the experiencing organism; they have a natural potentiality for learning. Rogers (1959, p. 5) describes the elements involved in significant learning as follows:

> *It has a quality of personal involvement.* The whole person in both his feeling and cognitive aspects being in the learning event. *It is self-initiated.* Even when the impetus or stimulus comes from the outside, the sense of discovery, of reaching out, of grasping and comprehending, comes from within. *It is pervasive.* It makes a difference in the behavior, attitudes, perhaps even

the personality of the learner. *It is evaluated by the learner.* He knows whether it is meeting his need, whether it leads toward what he wants to know, whether it illuminates the dark area of ignorance he is experiencing. The locus of evaluation, we might say, resides definitely in the learner. *Its essence is meaning.* When such learning takes place, the elements of meaning to the learner is built into the whole experience.

Therefore, meaningful learning is basically self-directed and is a matter of self-responsibility. This type of learning is individualized and significant. Learners define their learning needs and the instructor facilitates their learning.

Principles of Learning

Theories of learning are of use only if they are applied to the facilitation of learning. Hilgard and Bower (1966, pp. 562–564) identified principles from the three categories of learning theories.

A.   Principles emphasized in S–R theory (behaviorism):

1. The learner should be active, rather than a passive listener or viewer.
2. Frequency of repetition is important in acquiring skill such as typing, playing the piano, or speaking a foreign language.
3. Reinforcement is important, that is, desirable or correct responses should be rewarded.
4. Motivational conditions are important for learning.
5. Conflicts and frustrations in learning situations must be recognized and provision must be made for their resolution or accommodation.

B.   Principles emphasized in cognitive theory:

1. Learning problems should be presented in a way that their structure and interrelatedness is clear to the learner.
2. The organization of content is an important factor in learning and is an essential concern of the curriculum planner.
3. Learning with understanding is more permanent and more transferable than rote learning or learning by formula.
4. Goal-setting by the learner is important; motivation for learning, successes and failures determine which future goals are set.
5. Divergent thinking, which leads to inventive problem solving or the creation of novel and valued products, is to be nurtured along with convergent thinking, which leads to logically correct answers.

C.   Principles from motivation and personality theory (humanism):

1. The learners' abilities are important, and provisions should be made for different abilities.

2. The learner should be understood in terms of the influences that have shaped the unique development each individual has experienced.

3. The anxiety level of the individual learner is a factor affecting learning. With some kinds of tasks, high-anxiety learners perform better if not reminded of how well or poorly they are doing, while low-anxiety learners do better when interrupted with comments on their progress.

4. The organization of motives within the individual is a factor that influences learning.

5. The group atmosphere of learning (competition vs. cooperation, authoritarianism vs. democracy, individual isolation vs. group identification) will affect satisfaction in learning as well as the products of learning.

CONCEPT OF MARGIN

A theory relating to adult learning is called "differential psychology of the adult" developed by McClusky. He proposes the S–O–R formula: stimulus–person (adult)–response. This is an expression of the S–R theory (stimulus–response) of the behaviorists to include O, the intervening variable (the one being stimulated and responding). He states that the person (O) is the unique entity in a learning situation. Perception, which is organized and highly selective, influences the importance of the O. Persons perceive things in patterns that are meaningful to them. Not only is there selective exposure, but within the exposure field, there is also selective awareness (McClusky, 1970, p. 81).

McClusky sees learning as not only elaborate exchanges among stimuli, responses, and learners, but also as a dynamic process. One approach to looking at adult learning is to understand the concept of margin. He explains (1970, p. 82):

> Margin is a function of the relationship of Load to Power. In simplest terms, Margin is surplus Power. It is the Power available to a person over and beyond that required to handle this Load. By Load we mean the demands made on a person by self and society. By Power we mean the resources, i.e. abilities, possessions, position, allies, etc., which a person can command in coping with Load. Margin may be increased by reducing Load or increasing Power, or it may be decreased by increasing Load and/or reducing Power. We can control both by modifying either Power or Load. When Load continually matches or exceeds Power and if both are fixed and/or out of control, or irreversible, the situation becomes highly vulnerable and susceptible to breakdown. If, however, Load and Power can be controlled, and better yet, if a person is able to lay hold of a reserve (Margin) of Power, he is better equipped to meet unforeseen emergencies, is better positioned to take risks, can engage in exploratory, creative activities, is more likely to learn, etc., i.e., do those things that enable him to live about a plateau of mere self-subsistence.

Your margin is the surplus of your power over your load. Power is all your abilities and the resources that you possess to help you manage the tasks of living. These factors consist of your physical, intellectual, social, and economic abilities and are the tools you use to deal with your load. Load refers to the demands placed upon you. External load includes your obligations created by various social roles, for example, wife, mother, nurse, student. Internal load could be viewed as the expectations you impose upon yourself, such as the need to excel or the need to succeed (Gessner, 1979, p. 30). If your responsibilities (load) are equal to or greater than your capabilities (power), you have no margin and may have difficulties functioning effectively. However, when your power is greater than your load, you have developed a surplus of power and, therefore, have margin. Having this margin allows you to be creative, to learn, to deal with stress, or to undertake new challenges such as returning to school (Gessner, 1979, p. 31). The amount of power that you have determines your level and range of performance. The surplus (margin) indicated by your load/power ratio that can be applied to achievement is most important to the image that you have of yourself.

You might want to take a few moments and reflect on this concept of margin. What constitutes your load and your power? What responsibilities do you have now? What resources and abilities do you have? How much margin do you have? How might your margin be increased? By decreasing your load, increasing your power, or a combination of both?

ANDRAGOGY

In discussing his theory of how adults learn, Knowles used the term "andragogy" (the art and science of helping adults learn) versus pedagogy (the art and science of teaching children). Even though there is controversy about andragogy (see Cross, 1981; Elias, 1979; Carlson, 1979), it would be useful for you to have an understanding of the four assumptions about the characteristics of adult learners that are different from the assumptions about child learners. Knowles (1970, p. 39) describes these assumptions as follows:

> As a person matures, (1) his self-concept moves from one of being a dependent personality toward one of being a self-directing human being; (2) he accumulates a growing reservoir of experience that becomes an increasing resource for learning; (3) his readiness to learn becomes oriented increasingly

to the developmental tasks of his social roles; and (4) his time perspective changes from one of postponed application of knowledge to immediacy of application, and accordingly his orientation toward learning shifts from one of subject-centeredness to one of problem-centeredness.

Each of the assumptions about pedagogy and andragogy will be briefly explained.

Self-Concept

Rogers defines self-concept or self-structure as "an organized configuration of perceptions of the self which are admissible to awareness" (1951, p. 501). Your self-concept is composed of such elements as the perceptions of your characteristics and abilities, the perceptions and concepts that you have of yourself in relation to others and to your environment, the values that you perceive as associated with your experiences and objectives, and the goals and ideals that you perceive as having positive or negative valence (Rogers, 1951, p. 501).

Knowles states that as you grow and mature your self-concept moves from one of total dependency (the infant) to one of increasing self-directedness. He continues (1970, p. 55),

> Andragogy assumes that the point at which an individual achieves a self-concept of essential self-direction is the point at which he psychologically becomes adult. A very critical thing happens when this occurs: the individual develops a deep psychological need to be perceived by others as being self-directed. Thus, when he finds himself in a situation in which he is not allowed to be self-directing, he experiences a tension between that situation and his self-concept (how he perceives himself). His reaction is bound to be tainted with resentment and resistance.

Knowles, then, believes that adults have the need to be self-directing, to be treated with respect, to make their own decisions, and to be seen as unique human beings. They resist learning under conditions that are not congruent with their self-concept as autonomous individuals (Knowles, 1970, p. 40).

Experience

Adults have a reservoir of life experiences. Kidd mentions three related notions in comparing experiences of children and adults: (1) adults have more experiences, (2) adults have different kinds of experiences, and

(3) adult experiences are organized differently from those of children (Kidd, 1973, p. 46). To adults, they *are* their experiences. The accumulated experiences define who the adult is; a set of unique experiences establishes a self-identity (Knowles, 1970, p. 44). Because of this, adults have deep investment in the value of their experiences.

These differences in experience between children and adults have various consequences for learning: (1) adults have more to contribute to the learning, (2) adults have a rich foundation of experiences that can relate to new experiences, and (3) adults have acquired a large number of fixed habits and patterns of thought and, therefore, may be less open-minded (Knowles, 1970, p. 44). You have accumulated a great volume and variety of experiences on which to base your new learning. However, you may find that creative thinking and innovation may be somewhat difficult for you because of the habits and opinions you have already formed.

Readiness to Learn

Adults develop their readiness to learn as a result of the developmental tasks and requirements of various social roles. In another chapter you will read about adult development and life stages. Much of the learning that you do is related to the various tasks or roles that you perform. You are now returning to school to continue your formal nursing education. You are "ready to learn" additional information and develop new values as you prepare yourself for a new professional role.

Orientation to Learning

You enter into education now with a different time perspective than you had as a child; this has an impact upon the way you view learning. You want to apply immediately what you learn today, that is, you have a "perspective of immediacy of application toward most of your learning" (Knowles, 1970, p. 48). Adults' learning is usually problem centered or purpose centered.

Have you thought that you, as an adult, take part in an educational activity (your current one or a previous continuing education activity) because you are experiencing some inadequacy in coping with your current life or work situation? Is this a reason why you are returning to school, to prepare yourself to cope more effectively with your work? "To adults, education is a process of improving their ability to deal with life problems they face now. They tend, therefore, to enter an educational activity in a problem-centered frame of mind" (Knowles, 1970, p. 48).

CHARACTERISTICS OF ADULT
LEARNERS: A MODEL

Cross offers a framework that accommodates current knowledge about what is known about adults as learners. The CAL model (characteristics of adult learners) consists of two classes of variables: (1) personal characteristics that describe the learners, and (2) situational characteristics that describe the conditions under which learning takes place. The personal characteristics represent the gradual growth of children into adults. Three dimensions are included: physical, psychological, and sociocultural. The situational characteristics differentiate the adult education from education for children; adults are usually part-time learners and they are normally volunteers. The situational variables of the CAL model are usually expressed as dichotomies: part-time versus full-time learning, and voluntary versus compulsory learning (Cross, 1981, p. 235).

However, neither part-time versus full-time learning nor voluntary versus compulsory learning are actually true dichotomies. You, as a nurse, take part in many continuing education activities on a part-time basis voluntarily. Now you may be continuing your formal nursing education part time, but at some point in the future you may return to school full time. And for many nurses today, continuing education is mandated for relicensure, which is not exactly voluntary! In general, however, most adult learning is part time and voluntary.

It would appear that Cross's CAL model incorporates many existing theories of adult learning and characteristics of adults into a common framework. "It does provide a mechanism for thinking about a growing, developing human being in the context of the special situations common to part-time volunteer learners" (Cross, 1981, p. 243). Some of the assumptions of andragogy can be incorporated into the CAL model. For example, readiness to learn would probably be largely a function of the sociocultural continuum of life phases. And self-concept would be aligned with the psychological dimension (Cross, 1981, p. 238).

USING YOUR KNOWLEDGE
OF ADULT LEARNERS

In this chapter several learning theories and characteristics of adults have been reviewed. Although, as a group, nurses returning to school have similarities, remember that you are a unique person. You, as an adult, can learn and you can use your knowledge of adult learning to increase your successes while in school.

As you experience school, keep in mind the following points and consciously apply them to your situation:

1.   *Need to learn.* Adult learners must feel a need to learn. They need to perceive the goals of the educational experience as their goals. This problem-centered learning situation helps to motivate them to seek solutions or to better understand the need to learn. Are you certain that you feel a need to learn? If you don't, perhaps now is not the best time for you to return to school.

2.   *Previous experiences.* Adults have had many experiences, and their current learning experiences need to relate to these previous ones. In other words, your previous experiences, at work or at school, can be used as bases for your new learning. Don't expect your school experiences now to be the same as your prior experiences, but think through ways in which they are similar.

3.   *Practicality.* Adult learners are practical and seek solutions to problems. Their learning experiences should articulate as closely as possible with their immediate needs and goals. You should express your needs and problems to your instructor. Learning activities, such as case studies, role playing, and small group work, which present problems and settings similar to those you actually face, can be incorporated into your studies. These situations may assist you in determining practical solutions to your problems.

4.   *Learner involvement.* Adult learners need to be involved in planning, implementing, and evaluating their learning experiences. "If the goals of the learning opportunity are to relate to the needs and problems of the learner, then the search for solutions must be undertaken with the learners. In the process, the learner will be able to influence the goals and learn the process of problem solving" (Boyle, 1981, pp. 210–211). This means that you should express your desires to the faculty. Be realistic; if you are enrolled in a community health course, you are going to have to study community health. However, you may be able to explore in depth a certain aspect that relates to your long-term interest. The faculty member may be very willing to modify the course activities to accommodate your special interests and needs.

5.   *Self-concept.* Adult learners have the need to see themselves as being essentially self-directing and to be perceived by others as being self-directing. Because of this need, you desire to be treated with respect and to make your own decisions. You will resent situations when you are treated like a child. Being self-directing also means you have to assume responsibility for your own learning. This may be difficult for you because you may not have been exposed to self-directed learning. Don't be hesitant to ask questions to clarify your responsibilities.

6.   *Feedback.* Adult learners should seek feedback so that they can evaluate their success in reaching their goals. Success in reaching

their goals is necessary to maintain their motivation in learning (Boyle, 1981, p. 211). The instructor will have planned several methods for evaluating your performance. Tests, papers, role playing, clinical performance, or class presentations are common ways of evaluating a student and providing feedback on meeting the learning goals. You could suggest additional ways for getting feedback if your goals are somewhat different than those of others in the class. Perhaps you could arrange for several short conferences with your instructor. Maybe keeping a journal about your thoughts and insights will give you a means of feedback on the quality of your learning experiences.

Summary

It must be remembered that characteristics of adult learners and the principles of adult learning are just now becoming influential in determining practices in higher education. Many of your instructors will teach using the methods that were prominent when they themselves were students, which did not include many of the principles discussed in this chapter. Be understanding. Realize you may know something that your instructors do not know or do not put into practice. You can learn, and together you, your colleagues, and your instructors can have meaningful learning experiences.

REFERENCES

Boyle, Patrick G. *Planning Better Programs*. New York: McGraw-Hill Book Co., 1981.

Carlson, Robert A. "The Time of Andragogy," *Adult Education*, 29, no. 5 (Fall 1979), pp. 53–57.

Cross, K. Patricia. *Adults as Learners*. Reprinted by permission of Jossey-Bass, Inc., San Francisco, 1981.

Dubin, Samuel S., and Morris Okun. "Implications of Learning Theories for Adult Instruction," *Adult Education*, 24, no. 1 (1973), pp. 3–19.

Elias, John L. "Andragogy Revisited," *Adult Education*, 29, no. 4 (Summer 1979), pp. 252–255.

Gessner, Barbara A. "McClusky's Concept of Margin," *Journal of Continuing Education in Nursing*, 10, no. 2 (March–April 1979), pp. 30–33.

Hilgard, Ernest R., and Gordon H. Bower. *Theories of Learning*, 3rd ed. New York: Appleton-Century-Crofts, 1966.

Houle, Cyril O. *Continuing Your Education*. New York: McGraw-Hill Book Co., 1964.

———. *The Inquiring Mind*. Madison: University of Wisconsin Press, 1961.

Kidd, J. R. *How Adults Learn*, 2nd ed. New York: Association Press, 1973.

Knowles, Malcolm. *The Adult Learner: A Neglected Species*, 2nd ed. © 1978 by Gulf Publishing Co., Houston, Tex. Used by permission. All rights reserved.

———. *The Modern Practice of Adult Education: Andragogy Versus Pedagogy*. New York: Association Press, 1970.

Maslow, Abraham. *Motivation and Personality*. New York: Harper & Row, Pub., Inc. 1970.

———. *The Farther Reaches of Human Nature*. New York: Viking Press, 1971.

McClusky, Howard Y. "An Approach to a Differential Psychology of the Adult Potential," in *Adult Learning and Instruction*, ed. Stanley M. Grabowski. Washington, D.C.: Adult Education Association of U.S.A., 1970.

McKinnon, Joe W., and John W. Renner. "Are Colleges Concerned with Intellectual Development?" *American Journal of Physics*, 3, no. 9 (September 1971), pp. 1047–1053.

Milhollan, Frank, and Bill Forisha. *From Skinner to Rogers: Contrasting Approaches to Education*. Lincoln, Neb.: Professional Educators Publications, Inc., 1972.

Muzio, Lois G., and Julianne P. Ohashi. "The RN Student—Unique Characteristics, Unique Needs," *Nursing Outlook*, 27, no. 8 (August 1979), pp. 528–532.

Rogers, Carl R. *Client-Centered Therapy*. Boston: Houghton Mifflin Company, 1951.

———. *Freedom to Learn*. Columbus, Ohio: Charles E. Merrill Publishing Co., 1969.

Srinivasan, L. *Perspectives on Nonformal Adult Learning*. North Haven, Conn.: Van Dyck, 1977.

Tough, Allen. *The Adult's Learning Projects*, 2nd ed. Austin, Tex.: Learning Concepts, Inc., 1979.

Wadsworth, Barry J. *Piaget's Theory of Cognitive Development*, 2nd ed. New York: Longman, Inc., 1979.

12

Adult Development and Returning to School

Charlotte Abbink, R.N., M.S.N.

INTRODUCTION TO DEVELOPMENT

Me? But I'm an Adult!

Let's play a word-association game. What comes to mind when you read the word "development"—a new baby, a psychology course, Piaget, kids, your child's first step, learning problems, and on and on? What about *you*? Did you think about yourself and where *you* are in the process of development? Often development is a concept applied only to children. But actually it is a life-long process of sequential, orderly changes in one's physical, social, and emotional characteristics. This dynamic process is propelled by our continual efforts to create a comfortable fit between who we have been, who we are now, and who we want to become.

Researchers such as Daniel Levinson, Roger Gould, and Erik Erikson have proposed theories for understanding adult development. These theories are based on the premises that (1) development continues in definable, predictable patterns throughout life, (2) critical periods of physical and psychosocial reorganization occur when certain concerns and tasks become salient, and (3) each stage requires new learning in both the affective and cognitive domains to master current tasks that are foundational to future tasks.

A Conceptual Approach to Adult Development

Daniel Levinson has described one of the more comprehensive theories of adult development. Although this research was with men, Gail Sheehy has expanded the research to include women. Both Levinson and Sheehy present similar adult development theories that identify age-associated periods of stability and transition.

The basic construct in Levinson's (1978) theory is that of "individual life structure" (p. 41). This refers to the pattern of one's life at any point in time. Some aspects of the life structure are central, such as family, job, friends, or religion, because they are highly significant and strongly influence other choices made by the individual. Other elements, which are less critical and more readily changed, are considered as peripheral. When a component of the life structure changes, it will result in a reorganization of the overall structure. The more central that component is, the greater will be the impact of its change on the structure. For example, on a day-to-day basis, the war in Viet Nam may have been a peripheral component to the life structure of any given young man in the United States until the day he received his draft notice.

According to Levinson (1978), it is this life structure that is dynamic in adult development and undergoes predictable times of transition and stability. During transitions the individual evaluates his life structure and either redirects his goals and modifies his structure or reaffirms and strengthens his previous choices and structure. During the stable periods the individual builds on the goals and choices made during transition and maintains an intact structure in order to focus on and accomplish the tasks at hand.

What is the impetus that moves an adult from a stable state into a transition? As one progresses through adulthood, his own experiences and capacities dictate that he must make adjustments to himself and his environment. It is these internal urges or external events that motivate the individual to reevaluate his life. Some transitions are precipitated by predictable life occurrences such as moving away from home, marriage, or retirement. These are anticipated maturational changes that require life structure reorganization in order for the person to adapt. Unexpected life situations can also force life restructuring and rebuilding around different goals and activities. For example, the 24-year-old woman who is in a stable state, building on her career choice as a model, but becomes a quadraplegic in an accident will be thrust suddenly into a transitional state. In normal circumstances, she may not have been ready to reevaluate her life structure. She is now forced to do so.

The Levinson (1978) theory identifies ten age-linked stages in adult development. These stages are (1) early adult transition (age 17 to 22), (2) entering the adult world (age 22 to 28), (3) age thirty transition (age 29 to 33), (4) settling down (age 33 to 40), (5) the mid-life transition (age 40 to 45), (6) entering middle adulthood (age 45 to 50), (7) age fifty transition (age 50 to 55), (8) culmination of middle adulthood (age 55 to 60), (9) late adult transition (age 60 to 65), and (10) late adulthood (age 65 and older). Significant activities are associated with each stage and provide the opportunity for continued personal learning and growth.

ASSESSING DEVELOPMENTAL STATUS
AND RETURNING TO SCHOOL

How Did You Decide on Nursing?

Before considering the characteristics of each adult stage and their relationship to your educational and career mobility, you need to review your individual career development history, particularly your entrance into nursing. This is essential because a basic premise of the developmental process is that all preceding experiences and attitudes help shape current and future characteristics. Ask yourself these questions: How old was I when I started thinking about being a nurse? Were these thoughts based on fact or fantasy—maybe childhood fantasy? What initially motivated me toward being a nurse? Who had input into my earliest thoughts about nursing? For many nurses, the answers to these questions will take them back to childhood or adolescence. Some outstanding experience or special family member may have made an indelible impression about nurses or nursing. These impressions can ultimately become significant factors in the career choice and its value to you. Continue on with these questions: At what age did I make the initial major commitment to nursing, that is, decide this is the course of studies I will follow? How knowledgeable was I about the profession of nursing when I made this first commitment? How knowledgeable was I about myself as a working person, my skills, my likes and dislikes? Who had input into this decision? What professional career advice did I get? Among nurses, the initial career commitment is usually made either shortly after high school graduation or later as a mid-life second career choice after children are in school or have left home. This career decision, whether made as a young adult or in mid-life, is often strongly influenced by personal impressions of nursing that are based on very little factual information about the work. The decision may be made with minimal professional advice and limited experience as an employed person. After looking at your initial interests and motivations for entering nursing, you may get some feel for why being a nurse, as a part of your life structure, may undergo periods of stability and transition. At age 38 can you live with the decision made by an inexperienced 18-year-old, which was nurtured by an 8-year-old's fantasy?

The following discussion will give a brief description of the adult developmental stages according to Levinson's (1978) theory and the major corresponding career and educational concerns. The reader should keep in mind that these are generalizations that will have varying degrees of "fit" to your own life experiences.

Young Adult Transition   This life stage can be considered as a time of liberation and exploration. The relationships with family and institutions are being modified or terminated. New choices are being made that will foster the construction of an *initial* adult identity. To begin this process, the young person needs to be less dependent on family support and to have greater independence in decision making regarding living arrangements, activities, career preparation, jobs, and interpersonal relationships.

It is during this time that an initial career commitment is often made either by finding a job or by enrolling in preparatory courses for a career. Often this initial career choice is based on limited knowledge about what people working in that career do day by day. It is characteristic of this age group for the choice to be motivated by idealism and/or a response to external expectations. Many young people choose nursing as a career with a sincere humanitarian concern, but with exaggerated expectations of what they can do to "help people." Others enter nursing because of family traditions or expectations.

To establish oneself in a career or job, one must "try on" an identity related to people in that career. Because the personal adult identity and career identity are developing simultaneously, at this time of life, they often merge. The career identity becomes a part of the new adult identity. Therefore, success or lack of success in pursuing the career or the educational preparation necessary for the career may have serious consequences to the personal identity. A senior student who was having personal problems and needed to leave the nursing program exemplified this by saying, "I've got to come back and finish because I'm just now becoming comfortable that *I am a good nurse*." She was saying that she needs to be a nurse now because being a good nurse has become a part of *who* she is.

Recognizing how interwoven and precarious career and self-identity are during this transitional stage, we have a perspective to look at the problems posed to the educationally mobile young adult when returning to school. While accomplishing the transitional tasks, this young adult will have "tried on" an initial adult identity as a nurse and, if successful, will be feeling positive about the career choice and being a good nurse. When told by someone in the nursing system, or by an intrinsic urge that "you should return to school," the implication is that you are not as good or as complete a nurse as you could be. This shakes not only the weakly grounded identity as a nurse, which is based on limited experiences, but also the newly developing adult identity, which is tied into being a good nurse.

To cope with the challenge to identity that is precipitated by the suggestion that one should return to school, the young nurse may select from several alternatives, which include the following:

1. Deferring any decision about returning to school until later when the career direction is more certain.
2. Returning to school with some uncertainties, but being open minded to identity changes.
3. Returning to school, but feeling under pressure to do so and resisting any change in identity.
4. Determining not to return to school because of either not needing or not wanting the additional education or a changed nursing identity.

Entering the Adult World   Now comes the time for energy to be expended toward building on the relationships, career goals, values, and life-style choices that were made in the last stage. This is a period of mastery, self-control, idealism, optimism, and a sense of rightness about the direction life is going. Most endeavors are undertaken with the idea that self-will and boldness are the keys to success. This confidence is a reflection of the high energy levels and power a young adult experiences when leaving adolescence. This "self-arrogant" attitude is necessary to deal with the barriers to entering the adult world.

The early period of career establishment is very similar to the early school years. Productivity is now a life focus just as in Erikson's school-age stage of "industry versus inferiority." Also, feelings about productivity generalize to become feelings about self; that is, I am what I do or accomplish. In school-agers, this is seen in the pride they exude when showing mother or dad their school papers. In young adults, the manifestation of this characteristic is in the difficulty of separating criticism of work from criticism of self. In both children and young adults, there is also a strong reliance on external evaluations and rewards for measuring how well one is doing. During middle adulthood, there is a mellowing in this area, and the person develops a stronger intrinsic sense of self-worth and so relies less on reflected appraisals. Since productivity is an important component of self-esteem, failure to produce either academically or on the job is a threat to the young adult ego.

How do idealism, self-willfulness, and productivity affect the experiences of the educationally mobile young adult? Although this discussion is not exhaustive, it will present some common concerns.

First, nursing curricula usually present an "ideal" for nursing care.

This may be easily accepted by the student who has moved from one program to the next with limited job exposure in the real world of nursing. On the other hand, students who have worked a year or more before returning to school or who are currently experiencing the "reality shock" of nursing may be torn between the ideal and the real. They *want* to give the ideal care being taught, yet sense that they may not be able to do so, while remaining hopeful that it is possible. One student, age 25, who has worked several years in an ICU stated, "In returning to school, I entered the conflict of realism versus idealism. This astounded me . . . but as the semester went on, I realized idealism is good. If one accepts the reality of a situation, there is little possibility for change. Whereas, with idealism, there is a chance to incorporate change." This student is in a growth (but also stress) producing situation of beginning to know how to work in the real world, yet valuing the ideal, as would be expected for her life stage.

A frequent concern for those counseling educationally mobile young adults is the heavy home, work, and study schedules that are planned. Idealism and the attitude of "I can do it despite terrible odds" can lead to poor planning and a hesitancy to seek assistance or other alternatives when problems arise. The usual approach to a problem is to try harder and stay up later. One student, age 23, reported, "I've been having sleep disturbances, excessive fatigue . . . and bursts of anger because I have studied so hard. I just don't know what my problem is . . . but if I try enough I can do it." This full-time student was employed part-time and was a wife and mother running two households, because being in school necessitated her moving to the city during the week and returning home on weekends.

Balancing the role adjustments of home, job, and school is particularly stressful to the educationally mobile young adult. In all these roles, idealism must be tempered with realism, but not to the extent that the dream or the enthusiasm is lost. Many young adults find that balancing roles is difficult because they are strongly committed to each role and want to put their utmost into all of them. As a result, life becomes bound up by these demands, with very little time left for self and relaxation. This quickly leads to chronic fatigue and depression.

The Thirties Transition   Between the ages of 28 and 33, another transitional period is experienced. The life structure of the twenties is reevaluated. This transition may result in slight modifications and enrichment of the previous commitments and life built in the twenties. Or it may be a time for dramatic change if the previous commitments to mate, career, friends, or life-style are discarded and new commitments are made. By this time, one has begun to recognize that a reliance on personal willpower is not the solution for overcoming life circumstances and problems. Therefore, the choices being made in this transition are more reality oriented than those made in the young adult transition.

At this transitional stage, nurses who have been practicing for 7 to 10 years often find themselves bored with their jobs, frustrated by stagnation and the lack of real professional advancement, and disillusioned about the direction nursing is going. For some, the solution to this problem is as clear-cut as changing jobs in nursing and reconfirming the career choice with new vigor in a new job. For others, this problem is resolved by leaving nursing for another job or career. In the current generation of 28- to 33-year-old women, this transition period may involve reconsidering the state of childlessness. Nursing may be left in order to remain at home to raise a family. For the educationally mobile nurse, dissatisfaction with where one is or where one seems to be going in nursing is often the impetus for returning to school. Being dissatisfied with the status quo, a decision may be made to advance in nursing. One thirty-year-old student described her returning to school as "a maturational crisis that began 2 years ago. I had a good marriage, thoroughly enjoyed motherhood, and yet felt vaguely dissatisfied with myself. My work was satisfying, *but* did I want to be doing the same thing 10 or 20 years from now?"

How does being in the thirties transition affect the experience of returning to school? First, the decision to return to school is usually made after careful deliberation and may be made at considerable expense to other aspects of the life structure, particularly to home and family. The decision is usually strongly influenced by an internal urge to redirect the career. Because the student has given considerable thought to nursing as a career, the motivation for seeking additional education is both to advance nursing as a profession as well as to advance oneself as a nurse. This student generally has well-defined goals and expectations for what should be gained in the educational program. To meet these goals, the student will critically evaluate each step of the program in relation to these expectations. Often this student will want some flexibility in the program for self-directed experiences, where one's unique educational goals can be met. The student quoted previously had as her goal to become a family nurse practitioner. She was familiar with the FNP role and evaluated her learning experiences in the baccalaureate program according to how they would facilitate her acquiring that role.

Settling Down   Again there is a stable period between ages 33 to 40, when one builds on the choices made in the thirties transition. There is a high level of self-investment in whatever goals have been set. The individual wants to establish an order and stability in life with long-range plans. At this time it is very important to feel that one is contributing to society and establishing a place in the world. The thrust is to "make it now." The career orientation becomes directed toward attaining seniority and authority by moving into leadership positions.

Among nurses who have remained active in nursing, this period may be the beginning of a highly productive time of life. Women with families often experience increasing freedom from child care. They now have more flexibility and time to spend on developing their careers. There are now more opportunities to enter leadership positions and to develop creative ideas. Both leadership and creative output in a career require that one have time to devote to the career, as well as have accumulated necessary experiences in the career. During the late thirties, these two ingredients of career productivity, time and experience, come together so that one's contributions become more evident.

A student who was completing her baccalaureate degree described why she returned to school at this point in her life by saying, "In the past I have used nursing as a part-time thing. Now I feel that I need to show what I can really do with it [nursing]." Another student expressed a similar idea when she said, "Nursing has been just a job to bring in additional income. But now that my children are growing up, I don't want just a job; I want nursing to be a *career*." Both of these nurses were experiencing a subtle change in their attitudes about nursing. They had committed themselves to have nursing become more than a job. For these educationally mobile nurses, nursing was to become a career, and now was the time to demonstrate that they could make it. The motive for returning to school was to upgrade professional skills. Education becomes an active investment of energy into a career life structure that is perceived as stable.

The Mid-life Transition   This is probably the most discussed adult developmental stage. It is frequently referred to as the mid-life crisis. Although there is little consensus as to the age when mid-life crisis occurs, there is considerable agreement about the characteristics of this stage. Basic to this transition is a profound realization of a finite lifetime and the need to realign life goals in terms of the time left to live. There is an internalization process that directs the person to establish an identity from the inner self, rather than from external expectations and directions. Self-identity and authenticity are questioned as the individual becomes more attuned to himself. There is a new self-acceptance as one becomes more the person he "wants" to be, rather than the person he "should" be as defined in young adulthood. In conjunction with this deeper understanding of self, the life structures, including marriage, family, friendships, occupation, and social roles, are reappraised and renegotiated. This process may lead to varying degrees of life structure reorganization or a confirmation and continuation of the former life-style.

Just as there seems to be an internalized social clock by which we measure personal milestones throughout life, there is also a "career clock" that sets the pace for where we expect to be in a career at identified points in our lifetime. One who has had a continuous career history checks his own career clock during the mid-life transition to determine if he is on time or behind time in the expected career development. Based on these perceptions of timing, the career is reorganized and new goals are set. With the perspective of years left until retirement, it may become obvious that the young adult career goals were unrealistic. To set new, more realistic goals is a healthy approach to this occupational crisis.

For some individuals this is the time to change career commitments. They feel that if they do not make a change now, they will be unable to do so in the future. The strength to make such a change depends on the person's confidence in decision making and the available support systems and resources.

For the educationally mobile nurse, returning to school during the mid-life transition can provide the opportunity for redefining one's nursing role while gaining credentials and a new self-confidence to advance in the nursing world. With a more internalized sense of self-acceptance and knowing who one is, this becomes the time to pursue activities of choice, rather than to do those things that please others. For many women, the bright side of the "empty nest" is the opportunity to return to school and accomplish dreams that were set aside for childrearing. One educationally mobile nurse, who identified herself as being in the mid-life crisis said, "During my mid-life crisis, I am starting my career again in earnest. As I approach 45, my internal clock tells me I have approximately 15 years of productivity left. This [getting back into nursing] is something I really want to do for myself."

Returning to school during mid-life can be fraught with anxiety. A frequently expressed concern is for having become academically rusty during the long interim since last in school. Accompanying this concern is often a worry about having to compete with "younger, brighter" students. Underlying this worry is the myth that intelligence declines after 30. Recent data from longitudinal studies indicate little or no decline in general intelligence during adulthood, but rather a gradual improvement until age 50 and then stability until shortly before death (Kimmel, 1974, p. 159). Certain intellectual activities such as verbal comprehension, spatial perception, and formal reasoning actually improve during adulthood with the accumulation of experience and learning. Although many middle-aged adults fear becoming forgetful, this too is a myth in that no real decline in memory has been demonstrated until old age. The major problem in academic functioning that some middle-aged adults may experience is the matter of speed. Because of gradual neurologic decline and sensory deficits, such as changes in eyesight, some individuals may have trouble with tasks requiring quick performance. However, if allowed to perform without the pressure of hurrying, they readily overcome this problem. This has important implications when educationally mobile nurses are being taught and evaluated on new skills.

Entering Middle Adulthood   Following the mid-life transition, a new era is begun. The life structure is restabilized, and one sets out to enjoy the family, career, and friendship choices that are part of the reorganized life-style.

For many adults, these are the "payoff" years. There is a strong sense of interiority and self-approval as one experiences a time of maximal influence and best judgments. The career may be at its peak in terms of power, prestige, and income. Now the individual has reached a point in life where she is able to demonstrate wisdom and sound judgment as well as vision and innovation. A primary developmental task during middle age is to share one's knowledge and skills with the younger generation or to become a mentor to a younger associate. The occupation often provides the opportunity, either directly or indirectly, to leave something lasting for future generations.

Although our society seems to value youthfulness and to be youth oriented, we operationally value age and wisdom. This is apparent when looking at the ages of people who are in high decision-making positions at all levels of private enterprise and government. It is the "over-forty" group that holds the major responsibility, influence, and control in local, national, and international arenas. This may become even more evident as the average age of the population continues to go up. If one is experiencing peak career performance, work may be the pivot around which all other relationships and activities are ordered. When this happens, any job stress or dissatisfaction can have serious effects on physical and mental health. On the other hand, a sudden or insidious decline in health that hampers the ability to work will threaten job performance, satisfaction, and consequently self-esteem. Although at any age ill health will be detrimental to job satisfaction, it is particularly threatening in middle age because of the realization that there may not be enough time left to develop another career. Also the knowledge that employers may be less ready to hire people approaching retirement can add to the stress of middle-age career changes.

Returning to school after the mid-life transition is becoming more common. This author has a number of nurse friends and colleagues in this age group who are actively pursuing advanced degrees. It might be suggested that seeking advanced credentials after age 45 is more in accordance with cultural norms than seeking entry-level credentials. However, Weathersby (1978) notes that no matter what the life stage, the unifying characteristic of educationally mobile adults is an idea that for me "now is the time for this" (p. 20). There is an internal readiness for the selected educational experience even if it does not fit cultural expectations.

Applying Concepts to Your Experience

As an educationally mobile nurse, you need to consider where you are in the process of development, what developmental tasks are salient to you now, and how your career fits into achieving these tasks. Some important questions to answer for yourself are the following: What brought me to this point? Where was I developmentally in relation to my nursing career when I decided to continue my education? Why did I choose to return to school rather than to do something else in or outside of nursing? What goals am I currently setting for myself when I complete this part of my education? How realistic are these goals considering my total life structure? How will my life structure be modified and reorganized because of what I am doing now?

Stability, Transition, and the Educational Process   According to Weathersby (1978), there is a difference in how one utilizes an educational experience depending on the state of the life structure. Those individuals in a stable life period will return to school to build on current skills, that is, to improve what they are already doing. For the individual in transition, returning to school is a means of redirecting the career.

Although these may be the motivational reasons for returning to school, once back in school, most educationally mobile nurses consider themselves to be in a transitional stage because they are moving from one aspect of nursing toward another. One's nursing identity can no longer be completely grounded in the previous roles because you are being socialized into the future roles of nursing. To proceed through this transition successfully, one must be able to "pull up roots" from the old identity and "extend roots" into a new identity with new and often uncharted roles.

If one accepts the premise that being in an educational program places one in a transitional stage, then how much of what is being experienced emotionally can be related to transition? Stress and anxiety are experiences that are inherent to transitional states. With stress and anxiety come a myriad of emotional and cognitive consequences, including skewed perceptions, vulnerability to criticism, internalization of criticism, the need for increased amounts of external "strokes" (because people do not have the energy to provide their own strokes), and the need to make experiences more concrete in order to reduce the stress of abstraction, which is interpreted as vagueness. How do these consequences of transition effect you directly because you are in an educational program?

A basic component of the educational arena is critique or evaluation of the student's work. To learn, you need both positive and negative feedback on your work. If you receive only positive feedback, do you really learn? By definition, learning involves a change in behavior. Negative feedback may be necessary to get at the changes that need to be made for learning to occur. Here arises a problem. At a time when you are vulnerable to critique, may internalize criticism, and need more external positive strokes, you are in a system based on critique of your work that often includes negative feedback. Therefore, what an instructor may view as "constructive criticism" aimed at helping the student change a behavior may be internalized by the student as a criticism of self as a nurse. When negative feedback becomes internalized as negative criticism, various mechanisms will be called forth in the coping process. Unless the student and the faculty take time to understand what is happening, neither will be able to move on with the tasks of the educational process, and both will be frustrated in their attempts.

What do you do when you feel you are receiving little or no positive strokes? Some suggestions you might consider include actively seeking positive reinforcement from your instructors by talking with them about your needs. You might ask a direct question, such as "What do you see as my strengths?" Positive strokes can come from your family and peers; they too may need a direct question to stimulate verbalization of how good they feel about you. You can give yourself positive strokes by reviewing mentally the things you know you do well or by listing all your accomplishments for a day, week, or month. It is important that you separate what you *do* from who you *are*. Positive stroking becomes more apparent usually when this is done. You are able to respond to the positive interactions you engage in as a person (and feel gratified by these) while dealing with the negative messages directed toward your actions.

Although all students experience anxiety and may internalize criticism when their work receives negative feedback, this problem seems to be particularly acute for educationally mobile nurses. Probably the best understanding of this is found by looking at the role changes and the developmental life restructuring that is going on as a result of being educationally mobile. Although each life stage provides opportunities for learning, each transition places a person at risk (Weathersby, 1978). We must respond sensitively to those risks both individually and in the programs that are designed for educationally mobile nurses.

REFERENCES

Kimmel, D. C. *Adulthood and Aging.* New York: John Wiley & Sons, Inc., 1974.

Levinson, Daniel J., et al. *The Seasons of a Man's Life.* © 1978 by Daniel J. Levinson. Reprinted by permission of Alfred A. Knopf, Inc., New York, and The Sterling Lord Agency, Inc.

Weathersby, R. "Life Stages and Learning Interests," *Current Issues in Higher Education* (1978), pp. 19–25.

13

Understanding Evaluation as a Part of the Learning Process

Helen A. Hamilton, R.N., M.S.N.,
and Martha A. Albert, Ph.D.

It is evident that returning to school can be a rather stressful experience relative to self-concept, role change, and professional competence issues. Once again you will be faced with having to prove your level of nursing knowledge and expertise via the evaluation process. Evaluation is generally fraught with tension for all involved parties: students, professors, administrators, accrediting agencies, and even employers.

In nursing schools, the evaluation process will consist of both written and clinical performance examinations. Written examinations are basically designed to measure your ability to recall key facts, concepts, and pieces of nursing knowledge. This is called "cognitive" knowledge, because it involves the thinking process. Nursing written examinations frequently are built around hypothetical clinical situations, and are written to measure your ability to make clinical judgments, assess clinical situations, and select appropriate nursing interventions. Students are prone to complain that written evaluations are selective, subjective, and biased. In addition, many nurses believe that the state board examinations identify competent practitioners, and they resent having to take further nursing tests for admission and/or advanced placement in a nursing school. Some nurses further contend that written tests cannot measure the interpersonal aspects of nursing—care and compassion. Although many of these complaints may be true, professors and higher education administrators view examinations as evidence of adherence to academic standards, a means of securing and maintaining accreditation, and a necessity for knowing at what curriculum level a student should be placed at any given time. The identification of different student levels based upon education or experience may be crucial for student success in later courses.

In addition to identifying what cognitive level the student is at relative to a particular nursing curriculum, it is also necessary to identify or validate clinical functional levels or expertise. The clinical performance examination is utilized as a means of identifying the student's ability to apply nursing knowledge in an actual clinical situation. Such an examination is not designed to prove whether you are competent enough to be a licensed professional. It is primarily used to measure whether or not you have mastered critical nursing content that will enable you to perform safely and at a higher cognitive level in clinical situations. It allows professors to identify individual learning needs of students so that the educational process can be tailored to meet those needs.

Is evaluation ever fair? This philosophical question has been raised by generations of nursing and nonnursing students. Examinations sample the students' knowledge or behavior and are used by administering organizations to make decisions about admission, placement, progression, and graduation. Since content to be sampled and high (or passing) scores may be arbitrarily defined, all testing standards are, in the final analysis, subjective. Nevertheless, they are based upon the best judgments of professional educators and most of the time represent those aspects of nursing knowledge and behavior considered important.

In view of the importance of evaluation to the learning process, the returning nurse must identify and utilize effective methods of coping with it. To do this, the relationship of the following factors to performance level and self-concept must be understood: (1) test and life anxiety, (2) study habits, and (3) test-taking skills.

TEST ANXIETY
AND LIFE ANXIETY

Test anxiety is one of the strongest deterrents to successful performance on any examination because it blocks one's ability to utilize cognitive processes effectively. Major sources of test anxiety include fear of the unknown, low self-confidence, perfectionism, lack of preparation, and the need to please others. For the returning-to-school nurse, anxiety may be derived from a number of these sources. Coping with the problem requires you to recognize the source and take positive steps to alleviate it.

Reactions to written and/or clinical performance exams may range from intense outrage to fear of failure. These reactions may be derived from the inevitable insecurity about returning to school or the belief that, based upon clinical practice and past education, you have already proved yourself to be a competent practitioner. Thus the evaluation process may be most anxiety provoking because you may perceive your professional competence is at stake.

"Will I be labeled a poor nurse?" "Am I really adequate?" "Will I be humiliated by having to prove I am worthy of further education?" Such questions reflect feelings of insecurity. However, the fact that you are fully licensed and are functioning at a competent level in your work setting should give you a sense of security. Answers to these "insecurity" questions can be based upon past experiences relative to your knowledge and skills as a clinical practitioner.

In coping with your feelings, it is important to realize that the riskiness that you feel is to your self-concept, not to your career. An underlying demand for self-perfection and a need to obtain approval from authority figures are common. However, there is the risk of setting unrealistic standards for yourself by expecting yourself to perform perfectly on all aspects of examinations. Such high standards can be self-defeating for several reasons.

First, you are really most interested in an education, not merely a "piece of paper." It is necessary to know whether you need additional work in a particular subject area. Second, failing to obtain as much advanced credit as you wish or having to take remedial courses does not negate your present level of competency. These are indicators that more knowledge and skills are required to attain the advanced level of performance to which you aspire. Third, no one expects you to know it all—except, perhaps, yourself. It takes courage to admit the need for remedial work or the necessity to enroll without much advance credit. Fourth, you may still believe that exams unfairly measure your ability. But, ultimately, it is your decision to be open minded about exams, recognizing their fallibility and potential value.

Burdening the educational experience by carrying a "lunch bag" of grievances tends to create more anxiety and inevitably interferes with the learning process. Therefore, if you are primarily interested in a high-quality educational experience and can accept the positive and negative aspects of the degree program, some of your anxiety can be alleviated. Understanding and accepting the evaluation process is a big step toward decreasing test anxiety. However, the problem may still exist as a result of "life anxiety."

Life anxiety relates to the many personal stressors that may produce physical and emotional overload. Usually this overload is a consequence of accumulated burdens, each of which seemed legitimate when accepted. If test anxiety is related to life anxiety, it can only be alleviated by reducing responsibilities. Unfortunately, it is not unusual for nurses to feel guilty about reducing their many responsibilities. Nurses often take for granted a state of task overload in their private lives.

Returning to school, with its resultant time demands, will require you to redistribute some previous responsibilities, set limits on extracurricular activities, and develop an organized study-and-work plan. To utilize your time and energy efficiently and effectively, you will need to assertively renegotiate some of your responsibilities with loved ones and the groups in which you participate. Avoiding life overload takes planning and careful thought.

When test anxiety is related to your personal fear of failure, it is important to recognize and learn effective methods of coping with it. This form of test anxiety can be identified by the following signs:

1. Inability to concentrate on studies.
2. Worrying weeks in advance about an exam.
3. During the examination, worrying about failing and wondering what will happen if you do.
4. Inability to comprehend questions on the exam or to follow verbal instructions.
5. Postponement of studying until the last possible moment.
6. Physical symptoms such as hyperventilation, dizziness, heart palpitations, or nausea during the examination.

Some methods of coping with this type of anxiety have proved effective. Relaxation technique involves an isometriclike tensing and relaxing of all muscle groups in the body. This exercise enables you to experience total relaxation and to detect areas of tension in your body. With practice you will learn to control your physical response to anxiety. If you practice daily, this technique can be effective in the actual testing situation.

Meditation, another means of coping with test anxiety, allows you to become more "self-centered" and in conscious control of your body's areas of tension. The primary source of the relaxation response during meditation seems to be the deep, slow breathing that accompanies this technique.

Although these techniques can be useful, an improvement in your study habits may also lessen your test anxiety. Good study habits ensure thorough preparation and familiarity with the content to be tested by written examination. When preparing for clinical performance examinations, good study habits can also help you to plan your preparation systematically. To reduce your test anxiety before a clinical performance examination, be sure you become familiar with the criteria on which you will be evaluated, the list of skills you will be asked to demonstrate, all aspects of your assigned client's care, and the routine of the hospital unit on which you will work. Depending on the situation, these may be just some of the areas you will need to address.

In conclusion, test anxiety may be viewed as a response to a threat to your self-concept, as well as an inevitable outcome of life anxiety. Life anxiety is caused by professional and personal task overload. Assertiveness can be utilized to aid in the reduction of responsibilities. Returning to school with a minimum of stress requires the willingness to give priority to your own needs during the educational process.

STUDY HABITS

Developing good study habits is one way by which you can alleviate anxiety relative to the evaluation process. Since many demands may be placed on your time, the first step to efficient studying is the preparation of a study schedule. Study schedules are beneficial for the following reasons:

1. Available time is utilized more efficiently and in a more flexible manner.
2. An increased amount of work gets accomplished.
3. You learn more and perform better on examinations.
4. You are provided with the satisfactory feeling of being in control of your life.

When making a schedule, certain general principles should be applied (Pauk, 1974, p. 2):

1. Make productive use of each hour block of time.
2. Utilize daylight hours. "Research shows that each hour used for study during the day is equal to one and a half hours at night" (p. 22).
3. Study class notes after lecture classes. This enhances retention and understanding of material.
4. Plan according to priorities and avoid excess detail. Too much detail leads to a waste of time.
5. Study approximately two hours for every hour of class.
6. Plan one-hour blocks of time in which to study, followed by ten minutes for a break.

Types of Study Schedules

Pauk (1974) identifies five different types of schedules that may be useful. The type you choose to implement will depend on your personality, circumstances, and perceived need to become more organized.

The *master schedule* is a schedule of fixed activities that needs to be drawn up only once a semester. On this schedule, you fill in all required classes, labs, work-related responsibilities, recreation activities, regular meetings, chores, or other fixed activities. Once these are accounted for, you will have an idea of where your free blocks of time will fall; these will be utilized for study purposes.

The *detailed weekly schedule* is an expansion of the master schedule. It can best be utilized when time demands are heavy and predictable. It too can be made once a semester.

The *assignment-oriented weekly schedule* is based on specific assignments. Half of the schedule identifies each course, the assignments and their due dates, and an estimate of the amount of time needed to complete the assignment. The other half of the schedule specifies the days of the week and the systematic plan developed for completing all the assignments within the week. This type of schedule may be useful in preparing for a clinical performance exam, as well as for preparing written assignments.

The *daily schedule* is planned for each day and is based on blocks of time available on the master schedule.

Long-term assignment schedules are used for assignments that span a month or more, such as research papers or projects. Accomplishing these tasks requires long-range planning so that you are not caught by the lack of adequate time to do a good job. Some time should be allotted daily for these assignments.

You may ask, "What difference does organization and planning make if you have no quiet place to study? Everybody in my family still expects me to be Mama while I'm home. Besides, I'm usually exhausted when I get home from work." It is true that, in addition to the formulation of a study schedule, good study habits also require conditions conducive to study. One such condition is a quiet, well-lighted physical environment. The library can be a good resource for study, especially during hours when you are on campus and are not in class. At home, a room must be designated as the study room. It should be relatively free from distractions such as pictures on the walls, novels on the desk, or any other items that could draw attention from your studies. The study room should also be well equipped with a desk or table, a comfortable well-padded chair, and up-to-date references materials such as medical and college dictionaries. Since one of the most serious obstacles to efficient study is noise, family members must be made aware of the times you will be studying so you can be accommodated. If you have young children, however, some negotiations and suitable arrangements will have to be made with your spouse and/or significant others. It may be necessary to plan more of your study time to take place at the library or at the times when your children are asleep.

If you are employed, try to study when you are most alert, which is usually before you go to work. Since you may not be able to utilize large blocks of time for study, it is important to identify ways you can use small, fragmented pieces of time, for example, during coffee breaks, as you drive to work, as you brush your teeth, or any other time you have available. The daily schedule listing things to do in order of priority may work best for you. Utilizing all available time will require you to have study materials in a format that can be transported from place to place. Cards may be clipped to mirrors or walls. Cassettes may be listened to as you do chores, drive to work, get dressed, or do other repetitious tasks. Being able to utilize the small pieces of time to study will give you more time to devote to all of your responsibilities.

Your general health is important to the process of studying and learning. It is necessary for you to maintain a balanced diet, get adequate sleep, and exercise regularly.

Your diet may determine the quality of your thinking ability. If your blood sugar is low, confused thinking, tension, and lassitude result. Protein is also valuable as a nutrient that supports efficient thought processes.

Inadequate sleep may lead to loss of memory, muscular tension, impaired comprehension of new material, and confusion. Therefore, avoid staying up all night to study. Develop a regular bedtime that enables you to get seven to nine hours of sleep each night. There may be times during studies when *sleepiness* becomes a problem and must be avoided so that you can complete a task. If this occurs, you might try the following (Pauk, 1974):

1. Take frequent five-minute breaks.
2. Pace the floor slowly while reading or reciting out loud.
3. Schedule recreation or academic assignments requiring physical activity at hours when you find it hard to study because of sleepiness. Most people tend to have sleepy periods at the same time each day.

Exercise enhances circulatory fitness and thus maintains body tone and mental alertness for efficient studying and thinking. Exercise should be planned for in your schedule.

As you can see, the development of your study habits can be rather complex. The key to successful studying is concentration and a positive attitude toward learning. If you utilize the information presented, your ability to concentrate on material to be learned will improve. The end result will be increased knowledge and decreased anxiety over the evaluation process.

TEST-TAKING SKILLS

Test taking can be a traumatic experience if you do not understand how to approach it. The first step, of course, is an understanding and knowledge of the material upon which you will be tested. However, acquiring this knowledge is not always enough to ensure success on exams if you lack adequate test-taking skills. The following are general principles of test taking that can be applied to most exams.

1. Get a good night's sleep and avoid getting involved in any recreational activity between the end of your studies and your bedtime. Such activity tends to cause an increased rate of forgetting recently learned material.

2. Arise early enough on the morning of the test so that you are not rushed. Have a well-balanced, leisurely breakfast.

3. Get to the examination site a few minutes early so that you can relax and clear your head of any stress-related thoughts.

4. Avoid discussing the material to be covered on the exam with other students. This tends to heighten anxiety.

5. Think positively. Your attitude will influence your success.

6. For the written exam, read directions and test questions carefully. Go over the test once and answer first the questions for which you know the answers.

7. Budget your time. Check periodically to see if you are making good progress. Allow for time to review your answers once the examination is completed.

To further enhance your test-taking skills, you need to be familiar with the following types of exams and some approaches to them: performance exams, oral exams, multiple-choice and written essay examinations, and true–false questions.

Do you know of any nurse who has not been worried by a clinical *performance exam* for admission to or progression within a nursing program? While performance testing may be threatening to your self-concept as a nurse, it is also a puzzle in terms of test taking. Skills for this type of exam are primarily of a preparatory nature. First, you need to become acquainted with the faculty examiner. Find out what the clinical objectives are and by what criteria you will be evaluated. It would be best to have this information in writing for easy reference and clarity. If possible, observe how the faculty examiner functions in clinical situations with other students and try to identify what his or her perspective is in relation to clinical functioning. Avoid listening to rumors about faculty in order to keep anxiety to a minimum. Second, familiarize yourself with the hospital unit to which you will be assigned for the examination. In most instances you will get a brief orientation, but this may not be enough to make you comfortable. Therefore, if possible, arrange to work with one of the nurses on the unit for a day or two in an observer capacity. This enables you to learn about the overall functioning of the unit, location of supplies, important policies, and key procedures that you may be called upon to perform. This information should help alleviate your anxiety.

Finally, find out about the type of client(s) you will be expected to provide care to and thoroughly prepare to deliver that care. As you proceed with the exam, try to remain calm and clearly focused on the tasks at hand. Even if you do not feel calm inside, attempt to convey the image of calmness. If you can treat the situation as if you were in your own work setting, you will probably feel more relaxed about it.

Oral exams may accompany the clinical exams. In the clinical situation you will not only be evaluated on your functional skills, but on your cognitive skills as well. You will need to be adept at responding to questions that address the theoretical basis for your actions and issues pertinent to the care of the particular client to whom you have been assigned. To prepare for this sort of exam, it may be helpful to have another nurse ask you various questions about your client's condition and nursing care. Oral exams are difficult because you have to articulate your responses clearly and understandably. It is best to think through your response for a moment so you can cover the essential points succinctly. Do not attempt to bluff your way through if you do not know the answer.

Multiple-choice exams are a form of written test that is very common in schools. The multiple-choice question usually consists of a short statement giving certain pieces of information, then a few words (known as the "stem") that set up the question, followed by four or five possible answers, only one of which is the correct answer; the remainder are called "distractors." Theoretically, multiple-choice questions should be easy because one should be able to choose the right answer through the process of elimination. However, a common mistake made with this type of question is that the question and possible answers are inadequately read. The directions for this type of exam generally tell the student to select the *best* answer; this means that there may be more than one "correct" statement. Consequently, there is a tendency to choose the first statement that seems correct without reading the remaining distractors. Another common problem is reading more into the question than is there. If you take each question at its face value and answer according to what is asked, you will perform better. Most questions are not written to trick you.

When reading through questions, concentrate on the main point, rather than the details. If you come across questions that are hard to understand, restate them in your own words. Helm (1981) has found that most students have a tendency to respond to multiple-choice questions by first reading the stem of the question, then reading the alternatives, and again repeating the process. Such an approach increases the student's anxiety level. She proposes that you cover up the alternatives, read the question, and generate your own set of possible answers. Once this is done, you then check the test alternatives. Through a process of comparative analysis, alternatives are selected or rejected. This strategy has proved effective because it (1) enhances understanding of the stem, (2) provides a systematic approach to decision making, (3) encourages productive thinking, and (4) increases the student's self-confidence.

After you have taken a few multiple-choice examinations given by the same professor, you may find that the questions and answers form an identifiable pattern. Your performance in this situation will probably improve dramatically as the semester progresses.

True–false questions can generally be deciphered by looking for partially false statements and for patterns of phrasing that are irrelevant to the subject area. It is important to try not to interpret a statement too closely, since most true–false questions are clearly stated. Do watch for words such as "always," "never," or "only" because these words usually render a statement false.

Essay tests require you first to read the question carefully in order to understand exactly what you are being asked. Words such as "discuss," "compare," "define," "contrast," or "analyze" will clarify what is expected. As you proceed with answering the question, use an organized approach and answer the question directly in the first sentence. The essay can then be developed from this sentence by utilizing facts and other supporting material. Since essay examinations seek to explore an overview of a subject, you need to have a basic understanding of that subject.

Skilled test taking requires an adequate knowledge base plus physical and emotional preparation. If you can utilize the principles and suggestions presented, you will improve your test-taking skills with each examination you take. Check your acquisition of test-taking skills by reviewing each exam you take with the instructor to determine your strengths and weaknesses in terms of content areas. At the same time, carefully analyze why you made an error. In many instances, errors are not made as a result of inadequate knowledge, but rather from an inability to take examinations skillfully.

CONCLUSIONS

Understanding evaluation means understanding its effects upon you. It means accepting the fact that the R.N. or L.P.N. behind your name means that you have met minimal safety standards; those letters do not automatically guarantee admission to schools or exemption from courses. You will be happiest in a program where you feel that you will be evaluated fairly. It is a good idea to investigate several programs to decide where you will fit best. The greater your respect for the evaluators, the more inclined you will be to accept their judgments about your performance. Also, the more familiar you are with the evaluation process, the better you will perform.

There are no tests of nursing knowledge or performance that have been consistently validated by nursing practice. Few performance measures have been shown to correlate with academic success. With all its imperfections, however, evaluation is a fact of life in academia where standards, however subjective, define the process from entrance to graduation. Your major tasks will be maintaining your self-confidence and effectively coping with the academic evaluation process with the least amount of stress possible.

REFERENCES

Helm, Phoebe. "Strategies for Success on Nursing Exams" (audiocassette). RN Tapes, Inc., 1981.

Pauk, Walter. *How to Study in College*. Boston: Houghton Mifflin Company, 1974.

Additional Resources

Crow, Lester, and Alice Crow. *How to Study: A Systematic Way to Learn, Pass Examinations and Get Better Grades*. New York: Collier Books, 1979.

Hanai, Laia. *The Study Game: How to Play and Win*. New York: Barnes & Noble Books, 1979.

Hopkins, Charles D., and Richard L. Antes. *Classroom Measurement and Evaluation*. Itasca, Ill.: F. E. Peacock Pub., Inc., 1978.

Richard, J. A. *A Student's Guide to Better Grades*. North Hollywood, Calif.: Wilshire Book Co., 1971.

14

*Orientations toward Professional Nursing: Traditional to Frontiering**

Katherine L. Jako, Ph.D.

Have you ever stopped to wonder exactly what it is that distinguishes the educationally mobile from the educationally immobile nurse? To be sure, the whole thrust of recent history in the profession at large, and within nursing education in particular, favors mobility. Yet each individual still makes a personal decision, weighing priorities and choosing among costs, benefits, and sacrifices. Consider the licensed practitioner without a baccalaureate degree. In the typical case, two or three years of basic preparation have been successfully completed; the state board examination has been faced and conquered; the letters R.N. now follow your signature; you have sought and procured gainful employment in your chosen field; as a member of the nursing profession, you willingly provide essential care and comfort to those whom you serve, and you find many aspects of your work satisfying and personally rewarding. Once engaged in the art and science of nursing, what is it that brings one such practitioner back into an educational setting, while another continues as before? If state certifications as an R.N., a safe practitioner, marks the *first* step toward a professional nursing career, what combination of personal, intellectual, and social attributes characterize the nurse who is both ready and able to take the *second* step? The title of this chapter contains a clue, "frontiering"; but to explain that concept and

*Research cited in this chapter was made possible by support from DHEW/Public Health Service Grant No. 5 DIO NU 29044, "The National Second Step Project." Substantial parts of the chapter were drawn from papers presented at two research conferences sponsored by the NSSP (Jako, 1980, 1981). Complete citations are included in the references.

how it relates to educational mobility in nursing, it will be necessary to set the stage with some background information.

Although the *idea* of postlicensure upper-division baccalaureate programs expressly designed for registered nurses had been taking shape since the turbulent 1960s, actual planning for the first accredited Second Step Program began in northern California in the fall of 1971. The climate in higher education was, in those days, receptive to innovation and open curriculum models. Spurred on by demands for more adequate health-care delivery systems, stimulated by the strivings of nurses for professional status, legitimized by governmental financing, and not unrelated to the rise of the women's movement, the idea became a reality at Sonoma State, a small university at the northern edge of the San Francisco Bay Area. Since then, as similar programs have proliferated throughout the nation, becoming less controversial and more established over time, educators have begun to view the Second Step phenomenon through the cool window of empirical research and to describe this unique student clientele.

During that same period of time, the nursing "press," in journals, conference reports, and pronouncements from the professional associations, has resounded with news of "expanded roles" in nursing. We tell ourselves that nurses are no longer defined as subservient care-givers, that they are moving into more creative roles, and becoming more autonomous decision makers, more enterprising, more "professional." Those of us who are involved in Second Step research have, no doubt, added to that clamor. Many of us feel that this particular educational model has made and is making an important contribution to the changes that are taking place. Our task has been to articulate the exact nature of that contribution and why it might be both theoretically and empirically linked with the premises and practices of Second Step nursing education. To that end, a number of studies have been conducted. Early investigations were single-campus studies conducted over the years from 1972 through 1978. More recently, the National Second Step Project (1978–1981) has utilized data from six diverse programs and a total of more than 2000 R.N. students. All analyses were carried out on the Sonoma State campus.

ORIGINS OF THE FRONTIERING CONCEPT

An externally funded research section has been an important component of the Sonoma State nursing department since its inception. When the very first students arrived in 1972, they were greeted with a barrage of data-collection tools, a curious form of greeting that has been maintained and supplemented. Data have also been collected from faculty, from students as they progressed *through* the program, from graduating seniors, and from graduates out in the field.

It was from one of those early postgraduate interviews with a student who had finished in the spring of 1974 (and was interviewed perhaps a year later) that one of the first bits of evidence bearing on this concept was collected. "Can you tell me," the interviewer asked, "why you entered the program in the first place?" This was the response:

> It was because the program actually sounded interesting to me. I think I had really reached a point in my own life where I was bored and restless, and I didn't know what I wanted. I had a lot of job dissatisfaction, a lot of things I saw going on in the medical world that I completely disapproved of; but you know, what are you going to do about it? And I really didn't have any monstrous plans. It just sounded exciting to me. Maybe I'm sort of a rebel or a frontier person in the first place.

At another point in the interview this same respondent, who was a school nurse at the time, said,

> I don't even know why I went into school nursing. I knew I didn't want to go back to that mechanical building where people are treated like machines. I knew there had to be another way to do it . . . . I feel that maybe the whole nursing program was a catalyst for me. I became tremendously interested in many, many areas that I had never thought about really ever before, that I had never even thought of being connected with nursing, or the medical world at all.

That is, of course, one interview with one graduate, a particularly articulate informant who, by describing what turned out to be a relatively common experience to which many other Sonoma students, graduates, and faculty members alluded less artfully, was perhaps responsible for our selection of the term "frontiering."

The next stage of conceptual development took place through a series of research seminars in 1975 and 1976. Based now upon a backlog of data and speculations, the "frontiering" concept began to be both broadened and refined. Two somewhat separable aspects of the "frontier" itself were discerned. Perhaps the clearest way of distinguishing the two is to think in territorial terms.

Picture a large map entitled "health-care delivery." Nursing inhabits a certain territory with two kinds of "borders." One is represented by a thick black line separating it from the adjoining territory, which is inhabited by physicians, and the other by an ill-defined, broken line, perhaps a range of mountains, separating it from a sparsely inhabited wilderness area. The central area of nursing's turf is safe and secure; it represents traditional and undisputed nursing roles—what nurses have always done, and what they continue to do well, the majority of the supporting roles of the health-care system, services for which demand is traditionally high and for which qualified personnel must continuously be supplied to meet that demand. Now move toward the borders—the frontiers.

The heavy line is, in a sense, a closed border. It can be thought of as an "issue frontier," where the issue is perhaps most succinctly expressed as one of control, the supremacy of the physician in all areas of health care. Recent history shows that the border between the two territories, while hotly contested and jealously guarded, is not impermeable. Passports can be arranged, for a price. Those pioneering on this frontier are nurses who perceive their roles not as taking something away from the physician, but as dividing up the responsibilities and action of health-care delivery in more subtle and discrete ways. In theory, if not always in practice, the roles of the nurse practitioner and the nurse clinician or specialist might be thought of in this context.

The broken line is thought of as an "open frontier"; in a sense it is less of a boundary than simply the "edge" of traditional nursing practice. The adjoining territory—"wilderness area" in terms of our imaginary map—is created by important gaps in the health-care delivery system, such as the increasing needs for preventive health maintenance, consumer advocacy, and psychosocial services for the patient. The path across the mountains may be unmarked and the positions on the other side may be ill defined, but the open frontier exists for the taking. Those who move toward it do nothing to undermine the traditional structure of health-care delivery, so its pioneers will use less energy in storming the gates against resistance, leaving more energy and time for exploration and expansion.

At this stage, let me remind you that no attempt to quantify or measure the concept had been made, although existing data on a great variety of topics produced findings that were logically consistent with the idea. For instance, to review only a few items, data from this one Second Step Program indicated the following:

1. The mean personality profile of students at entry was dominated by high scores on autonomy, a measure of liberal nonauthoritarian thinking and need for independence.

2. As they entered the program, about four out of ten of these students (42 percent) envisioned themselves as self-employed in their future careers, and even more (51 percent) were thinking along these lines as they graduated.

3. About a third of the entrants (32 percent) had selected the Sonoma State campus specifically because they wanted to parti-

cipate in an "experimental" program; and more than half (56 percent) indicated that their original choice of nursing as an occupation had been influenced by their perception of this field as one which "allows me to be creative and original."

4. When asked to view their chosen profession objectively, relatively few (36 percent) perceived it as one that was characterized by "originality and creativity," and that proportion was identical among both entrants and graduating seniors. But three out of four entrants and nine out of ten graduates endorsed that same phrase as one that was "important to me, personally."

5. Interest in the then new role of the nurse practitioner ran high. Among students who enrolled between 1972 and 1975, those who "definitely" aspired to become N.P.s took in a quarter of the entrants and more than a third of the graduates.

6. Finally, our data indicated that very early in their Second Step nursing education, almost two-thirds (63 percent) of the students reported that they had *changed* their ideas or developed *new* perspectives about the profession of nursing. Responses to that same question at the time of graduation approached unanimity: virtually all graduates (94 percent) reported such change—31 percent "some" and 63 percent "a lot."

What we had, then, was an idea, "frontiering," representing an orientation to nursing practice more or less characteristic of educationally mobile nurses who elected to enroll in a Second Step baccalaureate program. Next, we sought ways to "nail down" the concept in quantifiable terms such that both its prevalence and its relationship to other variables could be determined. To do so entailed a qualitative analysis of volunteered commentary from students in answer to a number of open-ended questions about why they had enrolled in the program, what they hoped to do after completing it, and their long-range plans for a nursing career. Points for frontiering were ascribed to a student who "shows interest in jobs that are nontraditional; questions established health-care delivery; is innovative and flexible in general orientation to nursing."

Almost half (49 percent) of the entering students were judged to show at least some evidence of this orientation; and for 38 percent, it was judged to be the dominant orientation. Their responses reflected a willingness to pioneer in or even to create new and more autonomous nursing roles. Many looked forward to functioning as independent practitioners, especially in remote or rural areas. Others hoped to "set up new programs, develop new ideas for health service organization," "work in the community as a consultant," "set up programs in mental health and nutrition, both the educational groups and for communities," "helping to provide health care where it is needed, being creative, innovative and constructive," "to joust with the system." Thus, our concept summarizes and names a cluster of attitudes that appear to be linked with an inclination toward certain kinds of nursing roles: specifically, roles that are less traditional and that will, if pursued, draw these nurses toward the frontiers of nursing practice.

Although this nontraditional bent was perhaps the most intriguing and illuminative of the orientations discerned among R.N. students of the early 1970s, it must be emphasized that it was by no means the *only* orientation expressed. About three-fifths of those nurses were headed in a variety of other directions: some aspired to professional leadership, some hoped for educational and/or research careers, and others were more interested in relatively traditional nursing positions. No single orientation was assumed to be inherently "more" or "less" professional than any other. Nonetheless, there was every indication that the men and women who are today seeking their careers in professional nursing are doing so on the basis of widely discrepant motivational structures. Along with "expanded roles," now an accepted term that has assumed a visible place in nursing rhetoric, comes an expanded clientele of potential applicants for these new roles. It is up to those of us who research the field to understand these new applicants—their perceptions of the profession and their aspirations, both of which will partially determine the contributions they will make. Frontiering, as presently conceptualized, is only one of several very legitimate orientations, *all* of which constitute fertile fields for further research.

TAKING A BROADER VIEW: THE NATIONAL SECOND STEP PROJECT

In the National Second Step Project (NSSP), the same kinds of qualitative data were collected from a much broader range of students: R.N.s entering six widely scattered programs in 1978 and 1979. In their own words, 693 incoming students responded to the following items:

> When did you decide to get a baccalaureate in nursing, and what were your circumstances at that time?
>
> For what reason(s) did you decide to get a baccalaureate in nursing?
>
> For what reasons did you choose this particular nursing program?

Do you have any special expectations of the nursing program in which you are enrolled? If so, what are they?

Describe briefly the position you would like to have after graduation.

What are your long-range plans for a position in nursing?

Since they were free to write in whatever they wished to say, there were many instances in which either *no* particular orientation could be clearly discerned or in which two or more orientations were expressed with equal emphasis. Such cases were eliminated from further analyses. Most, however, were consistent and unambiguous in their commentary. Five professional nursing orientations emerged from our analysis, all based upon the kinds of role expectations voluntarily expressed by entrants, and bearing upon their own futures in nursing: in-patient, community, vertical mobility, academic, and frontiering.

Two of these, the *in-patient* and the *community* orientations, indicate an inclination toward well-established nursing roles, each with its place in the history of nursing practice and tradition. Both are built around the *provision of service and care* for patients or clients, and the roles are played out within relatively conventional patient-care settings, which serve further to define those roles. One is the in-patient facility, whether acute or long term. Here the nurse provides direct care and service in a stable and relatively controlled environment. The other is the out-patient facility or community agency organization, whether public or private. Here, again, the nurse expects to provide care and service to patients or clients, but the practice setting itself is less structured. These nursing care activities may extend into the community, and the definition of "client" may extend to family, associates, and others. Yet the essence of the role is still the provision of service and care, and the manner in which care is provided is still controlled and further defined by the structure of the organization that employs and directs these nursing activities.

Those with a *vertical mobility* orientation have their sights set on *rising in the job hierarchy*. Most of these roles are probably, but not necessarily, played out in one of the conventional types of settings previously described. Yet the essence of the role is defined not in terms of its caring and serving function, but in terms of power relationships among providers of care, clients, and institutions broadly defined. Access to such authority may come either through promotions and seniority or through the possession of special expertise. Its hallmark is advancement, either through the institutional or the wider professional ranks of nursing. The expected role is one of influence and authority, regardless of the sphere in which it is exerted.

The *academic* orientation is fairly self-explanatory. It is built around the *acquisition and dissemination of knowledge*. Most of these nursing roles are played out on the terrain of the postsecondary educational institution or that part of professional nursing that is primarily concerned with education, research, publication, and academic advancement. In this "practice setting," nursing is more of an academic discipline than an activity. The prototype may be less interested in providing patient care than in teaching, conducting research, or perhaps promoting the status and respectability of academic nursing. The basic commodity is information or knowledge. Academic skills themselves are what the nurse hopes to market, not the nursing skills that an advanced degree may have provided.

The last orientation is still called *frontiering*. It is built around *movement into new areas of nursing responsibility*. Such roles are defined not by links with any particular type of practice setting, but by the manner in which the nurse expects to function. In general, the nurse expects to enjoy greater independence than is characteristic of traditional nursing roles. In some cases, these "new" roles involved relationships with patients or clients that have, in the past, been more typical of the physician's role, as in the role of the independent nurse practitioner. In other cases, role expectations are consciously grounded in a desire to change the profession, either by using nursing competence to promote the health of society or by improving the present health-care delivery system and the function of nursing within it. Because such roles are not yet well established, they often require the tastes and talents of the entrepreneur.

All five orientations were well represented among the sample of R.N.s ($n = 437$) whose responses could be clearly classified as they entered the six baccalaureate programs. Again, as in the earlier single-campus study, the frontiering orientation characterized the largest single group, 28 percent of the total. The academic and vertical mobility orientations occurred much less frequently (not quite 15 percent each), and the in-patient and community orientations each accounted for just over one-fifth of the total group, 21 and 22 percent, respectively.

Factor analysis of two large pools of attitudinal variables, one from entry and one from graduation data, served to further explain the five orientation groups, particularly in terms of their interrelationships. For instance, the in-patient orientation was fairly distinct from vertical mobility at entry. In the graduation data, these two orientations blend together. In other words, graduates who retain an interest in hospital nursing also tend to indicate ambitions for moving up in the hierarchy toward supervisory positions. Or, starting from the other end, you could say that many of those whose primary orientation was toward roles of influence and authority also, as graduates, tend to indicate an interest in remaining within the hospital setting and working their way up through the ranks. On the other hand, another route to influence and authority is by way of academia through acquiring additional expertise, knowledge, and credentials. Thus a similar blend occurs in the graduation data between academic and vertical mobility. Even the frontiering factor, which at entry was defined primarily by high interest in self-employment and in the nurse practitioner specialization, is at graduation much less clearly defined. It blends both with the community orientation, in terms of noninstitutional practice settings, and with the academic orientation, in terms of interests in being self-employed. A certain realignment of attitudes, preferences, and interests seems to take place during the course of the nurse's educational experience, one effect of which is that role expectations become more complex and less unidimensional.

Another lesson from factor analysis was that in terms of *attitudinal* data, the in-patient and the community orientations have very little in common. Both sets of role expectations are built around the provision of service and care, and both are clearly well within nursing's historically established domain. Yet items upholding many traditional perspectives on nursing roles and health care were positively correlated *only* with the in-patient orientation; correlations with the community orientation were either negligible or negative. Such outcomes indicate that if we want to call community health a "traditional" nursing specialization we can, but Second Step nursing students who are interested in those positions do not necessarily give evidence of "traditional" attitudes and interests.

Traditionalism in Expressed Orientation Toward Nursing Roles

These and other analyses clarified the ·nature of the orientations and how they relate to one another in terms of a theoretical dimension of traditionalism among Second Step nursing students. Frontiering still appears the *least* traditional, so they occupy the low point, followed by those with a community orientation. The in-patient group still appears the *most* traditional, so they occupy the high point, with vertical mobility adjacent. In the middle are the academics, who appear traditional in some ways and nontraditional in others.

This new dimension suggests once more that the total population of Second Step entrants veers slightly toward a nontraditional orientation. As shown in Table 14-1, half of these educationally mobile nurses were coded toward the low end of the scale, just over one-third toward the high end, and the remainder occupy the middle ground of academic nursing.

Table 14-1 TRADITIONALISM IN EXPRESSED ORIENTATION TOWARD NURSING ROLES

	Orientations at Entry	Total Population (%) ($n = 437$)
Traditionalism	Low: 1 = frontiering	27.9
	2 = community	22.0
	3 = academic	14.6
	4 = vertical mobility	14.9
	High: 5 = in-patient	20.6

DESCRIBING THE FIVE ORIENTATIONS: BACKGROUND AND PERSONALITY

Whether or not these five orientations can actually be said to constitute a dimension of traditionalism depends on what researchers call "construct validity." That is, once we have a body of data that claims to "measure" a certain concept, in this case traditionalism in orientation to nursing roles, we must find out how this measurement fits with other known factors. Do *other* known characteristics of the five groups form a coherent and interpretable portrait of each group, and are the five resulting "portraits" or profiles still compatible with the overall dimension of traditionalism? If so, what do these other factors add to our knowledge of traditionalism? Is it a useful concept? How does it help us to understand the nature of the educationally mobile nurse?

Much of the information in the next few pages is based on statistics, but don't give up! You may not know exactly what a statistician means by "significance," but for now just think of significance levels as operating in reverse, so to speak. Thus a finding that is cited at or below the "point on five" level (written as .05) is usually considered to be statistically significant, but anything *over* that (.06 or more) is *not* significant. On the other hand, when the significance level is a still tinier fraction (which could be anything from .04 down to .01 or .001 or even .0001), you can be increasingly certain of the statistical significance of that finding. The more zeros *after* the decimal point, the higher the level of significance.

We begin with a series of horizontal bar graphs, the first of which (Figure 14-1) shows four background and demographic variables. The question is, Do the orientation groups *differ* on these variables and, if

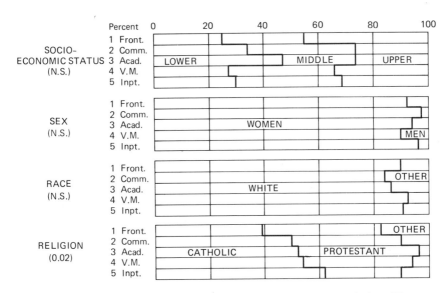

Figure 14-1 Four demographic variables in the study population. The first three show no significant differences in the five nursing orientation groups; only religion shows a significant difference. As the nursing orientation becomes more traditional, the number of Catholics increases.

so, at what level of significance? An N.S. (not significant) indicates that, using the chi-square statistic, differences among the *five* groups are not statistically significant, even though one group or another may stand out from the rest. Socioeconomic status, for instance, shows the frontiering group to come from a little *more* affluence and the academics from a little *less*, but overall the group differences are not significant. Sex and race differences are also negligible. Religious background, however, does differ significantly; the stair-step pattern of the Catholic responses suggests a linear relationship between Catholicism and traditionalism in nursing orientation.

Conventional wisdom derived from the social and political sciences tends to link traditionalism with age and nontraditionalism with youth. Figure 14-2 shows that Second Step student data not only fail to support that formulation, but they tend to confirm the opposite: a negative and linear relationship between age and the degree of traditionalism expressed (Pearson's $r = -.26$). More than half (53 percent) of the in-patient group enrolled at the age of 22 or less, compared to just a handful (8 percent) of the frontiering group. This single demographic fact has its effect upon other variables. Thus students in the more traditional orientations are far less likely to have married, and they probably earned an A.D.N. rather than a hospital diploma. As to the number of years between completing their basic nursing preparation and entering a

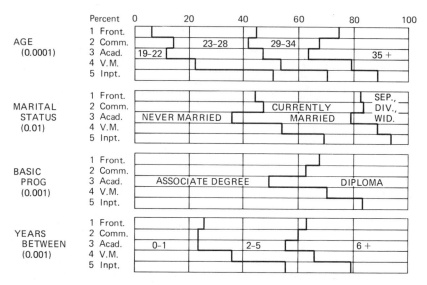

Figure 14-2 Effects of age on orientations toward nursing.

Second Step Program, here too we see a dramatic difference, with the time lapse being far shorter among the most traditional group. Note, however, that the academics tend to break up the linearity of these relationships: they include the *most* students over the age of 34, the *most* who are or have been married, the *most* who completed a hospital program, and the *most* with a lapse of six or more years between the basic and baccalaureate program.

Figure 14-3 shows only a handful of these students to have earned additional credentials or degrees prior to entry, and differences between the orientation groups are negligible. So in terms of "formal education," they are roughly equivalent. But when we look at *when* they made the decision to go for a baccalaureate, the in-patient group stands out sharply; most of them decided *before* being R.N.s, which no doubt affects the next variable: attendance pattern throughout their post-secondary education. Continuous enrollment is much more characteristic of the most traditional groups, but relatively rare for frontiering.

The next variable indicates whether these students, as they entered a Second Step Program, were members of professional nursing organizations. Again, the difference is significant and can be attributed in part to age differences. The traditionalists, who never intended to stop with an R.N. and who probably went straight from a basic to a baccalaureate program, are least likely to hold memberships, perhaps because they had not yet had as much time as the others to get involved. More than half of the frontiering group, on the other hand, having spent more time out of school, had joined these organizations and were already active members as they began their baccalaureate education.

212

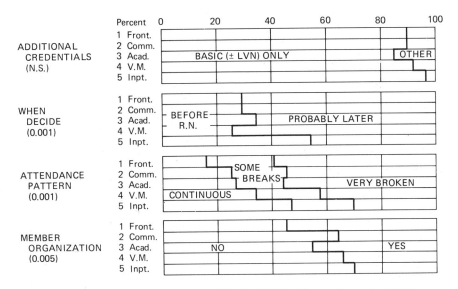

Figure 14-3 Four aspects of professional education and membership in professional organizations.

In terms of actual months of R.N. work experience prior to entry, Figure 14-4 simply confirms what all the preceding information would lead you to expect. Relatively few Second Step students, regardless of orientation, arrive with supervisory experience. Not many have experience in out-patient settings, but those that do are overrepresented among the *less* traditional groups. Experience in the hospital setting is

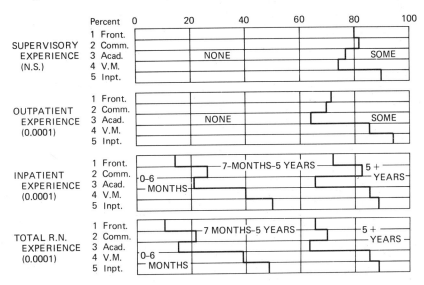

Figure 14-4 Four aspects of Registered Nurse work experience.

213

quite common, but again it is the traditionalists who tend to have only six months or less. Added together, you can see a clear negative relationship (Pearson's $r = -.27$) between R.N. work experience and traditionalism in nursing orientation. Among aspiring Second Step students, the traditional image of the angel of mercy, ministering efficiently but tenderly in a well-run hospital, seems to fade perceptibly as that environment becomes more familiar.

Figure 14-5 presents entirely different kinds of data, the mean personality profile of entering Second Step students. The basic question becomes, Do personality characteristics differ significantly by orientation group? According to scale scores from the Omnibus Personality Inventory (OPI), the answer is "Yes, in most cases." That is, on *each* of the fourteen personality characteristics measured by this instrument, statistical tests were used to compare the average scores of all five orientation groups with one another. Only on three "nonintellective" scales (social extroversion, altruism and masculinity–femininity) did the five groups score similarly. On the other eleven scales, listed next, significant differences occurred, suggesting that each orientation group has its own somewhat distinctive personality configuration.

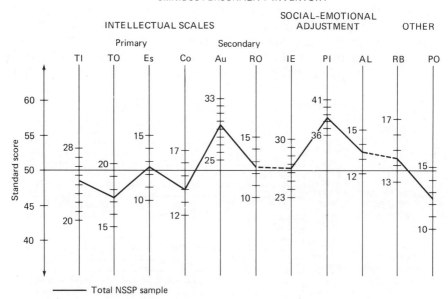

Figure 14-5 OPI profile for the total NSSP sample at entry (n = 786). This aggregate profile will be used to compare each of the five orientations toward nursing groups (see Figures 14–6 through 14–10).

Primary intellectual scales:	TI	(.01)	Thinking introversion
	TO	(.01)	Theoretical orientation
	Es	(.01)	Estheticism
	Co	(.01)	Complexity
Secondary intellectual scales:	Au	(.01)	Autonomy
	RO[a]	(.01)	Religious orientation
Non-intellective scales:	IE	(.01)	Impulse expression
	PI	(.04)	Personal integration
	AL[a]	(.04)	Anxiety level
	RB	(.01)	Response bias
	PO	(.01)	Practical outlook

[a]RO and AL are both scored in the reverse direction, so they actually measure religious *liberalism* (RO) and *lack* of anxiety (AL).

Here it should be noted, however, that the standardized mean for the OPI is based on data from a large sample of youngsters entering a wide variety of colleges and universities prior to 1962, most of whom were in their late teens. It still serves well as a stable reference point for viewing many diverse student populations. Yet in interpreting certain scales of social and emotional adjustment, such as anxiety level, it must be remembered that adolescence is typically an anxious period, especially among freshmen who are often living away from home for the first time. So when we say that our sample of postlicensure nurses, with an average age of 29 and a far more settled life-style, expresses only *slightly* less worry and anxiety than the average college freshman, we may also be saying that they are experiencing what amounts to a fairly high level of anxiety in comparison to their own peers in an adult population.

This brief presentation cannot do justice to the whole story on the Second Step student personality, but Figure 14-5 shows the basic outline as derived from the total of almost 800 respondents at entry, combining all orientations. All the subgroups will be a variation of this general "shape." Only those scale scores that differ significantly by orientation group are shown.

Two "peaks," for the total sample, are at roughly the same level. One is autonomy (Au) and the other personal integration (PI). At entry they appear to be remarkably independent, nonauthoritarian, and positively socialized. The rest of the scores hover reasonably close to the standardized mean—a bit low on both theoretical orientation (TO) and practical outlook (PO) and a bit high on anxiety level (AL), which is scored in the reverse direction and actually measures a *lack* of anxiety.

Now let's look at the orientation groups, going from the most to the least traditional. The traditional in-patient group (Figure 14-6),

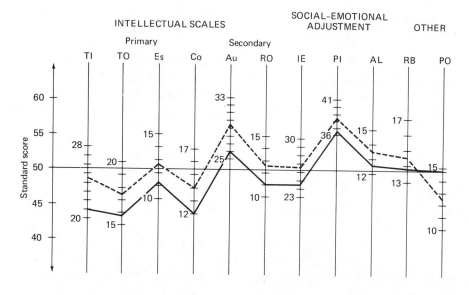

INTELLECTUAL SCALES   SOCIAL-EMOTIONAL ADJUSTMENT   OTHER

Primary   Secondary

Figure 14-6 Inpatient (n = 90) vs. total NSSP. This most traditional group is characterized mainly by low scores on the intellectual scales and a PO (practical outlook) score higher than the total NSSP sample.

——————— = Inpatient group

------------------- = Total NSSP

while still showing a modified version of the two peaks that we have come to associate with Second Step students in general, is characterized mainly by low scores on the primary intellectual scales: thinking and introversion (TI), measuring a liking for ideas and reflective thought; theoretical orientation (TO), measuring a taste for scientific thinking and problem solving; estheticism (Es), which taps artistic interests; and complexity (Co), which measures a flexible approach and tolerance of ambiguity. Religious orientation (RO) assesses religious liberalism, so they express *more* conventional religious beliefs and behaviors than do most Second Step students. Impulse expression (IE) shows them also to be more restrained, in spite of their youth; and AL indicates that they tend to express more worries and anxiety. RB stands for "response bias"; the easiest way to explain it is to think of it as measuring how much you, as a respondent, are out to "put your best foot forward" or to "make a good impression" on the OPI. Among the in-patient group, not very much. And the last one, practical outlook (PO), shows them to be about as pragmatic and utilitarian as most other college students. These may be very good nurses, well socialized and not excitable, but they will do best in relatively structured situations that do not demand a lot of abstract thinking and coping with ambiguities.

The profile for the vertical mobility group (Figure 14-7) is remarkably similar to that of the total NSSP population. Estheticism (Es) and complexity (Co) drop a bit below the overall mean, so they too show no particular fondness for artistic concerns or for novel situations and ambiguities. They are also less religious (RO) and a little more expressive (IE); and although their score on practicality (PO) is definitely lower than the in-patient group, they nonetheless are reasonably practical and down to earth in comparison to other Second Step students. The fact that this personality profile so closely parallels that of the total population prompts an interesting observation: The whole idea of the Second Step curricular model is closely linked with the idea of "career mobility." The congruence we see may suggest that students who are entering these programs tend, on the whole, to have personality characteristics very like this small, select group who actually verbalized the importance of "getting ahead" in the profession. So from our *observation* that the V.M. group is similar in personality to the total group, we can *hypothesize* that the "vertical mobility personality" seems to characterize

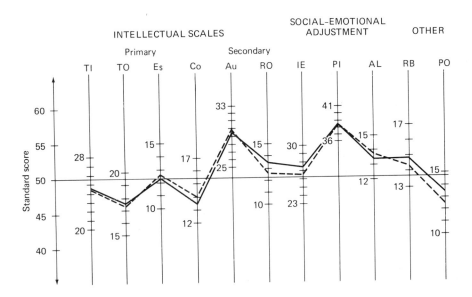

Figure 14-7 Vertical mobility (n = 64) vs. total NSSP. This group is remarkably similar to the total NSSP sample.

———————— = Vertical mobility group

--------------------- = Total NSSP

Second Step students in general. In other words, the kinds of students these programs are recruiting are those whose personality structures are compatible with a desire to move into positions of influence and authority.

The academics (Figure 14-8) display some interesting and interpretable similarities and differences. On three of the primary intellectual scales, they score considerably higher than the NSSP average, especially on theoretical orientation. They are definitely more intellectually disposed, although still close to the standardized mean of "college students" in general. But on complexity (Co), they are at about the same level as everyone else. They, too, are not fond of ambiguous situations where there is no clear "right" or "wrong" answer. The other place where they part company from the herd is in indicating a noticeable tendency, as a group, to want to "make a good impression"—the RB scale. This particular characteristic may indeed serve them very well in their academic pursuits, where self-effacing modesty has never gotten anyone very far. Along with this, we see a striking lack of anxiety and nervousness (AL), perhaps because as academic types entering academic

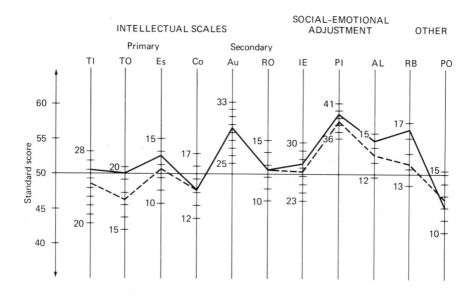

Figure 14-8 Academic (n = 61) vs. total NSSP. Predictably, the academic scores higher than the NSSP on three of the primary intellectual scales.

————————— = Academic group

----------------------- = Total NSSP

surroundings, they feel less threatened than others for whom the campus environment is one to be endured and gotten through rather than aspired to.

Figure 14-9 shows the community health personality, which is almost a caricature of the overall Second Step profile—the high points are higher and the low points are lower. TI, TO and Co are all a notch below the NSSP average, denoting at best only a moderate degree of intellectuality. On the positive side, however, there is a remarkably strong mean score on personal integration; they accept and embrace both themselves and people in the world around them. Emotional disturbance and social alienation are simply not to be found here. AL indicates that they are not worriers; and in this configuration, the relatively low score on impulse expression (IE) would be interpreted as an indication of being well controlled rather than impulsive or highly expressive, a trait that may serve them well in community health work.

The frontiering profile (Figure 14-10) is obviously the most elevated on all six of the intellectual scales, although it stands equal with

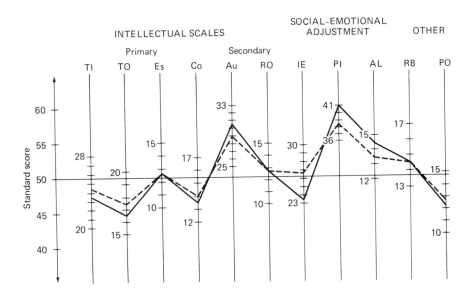

Figure 14-9 Community group (n = 93) vs. total NSSP. Note that when the NSSP total group score is low, the community group scores even lower; when the total NSSP group is above the mean, the community group scores even higher.

——————— = Community group

----------------- = Total NSSP

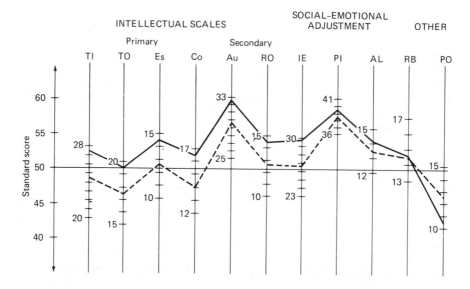

Figure 14-10 Frontiering (n = 117) vs. total NSSP. This group is the least traditional of the five groups. Note the high scores on the intellectual scales and complexity scale; the low score on practical outlook (PO) is also striking.

———————— = Frontiering group

-------------------- = Total NSSP

that of the academics on theoretical orientation (TO). The most striking contrast, however, is on complexity (Co), reflecting an experimental and flexible orientation rather than a fixed way of viewing and organizing phenomena. This particular trait is remarkably well adapted to the demands of frontiering nursing roles, which are by definition neither well established nor well defined. They also display the highest degree of autonomy (Au), combined with fewer religious constraints (RO) and greater expressiveness, imaginativeness, and impulsivity (IE). Finally, the PO score indicates relatively little regard for the practical approach and a certain devaluing of material possessions and concrete accomplishments. In short, they look very much like the adventurers that you would expect to find on the frontiers of nursing practice, and who might be marvelously unsuited to the regimented setting of a metropolitan hospital unit.

Finally, let's look at the two end-points on our dimension of traditionalism: the traditional in-patient versus the nontraditional frontiering orientation (Figure 14-11). The two personality profiles are totally

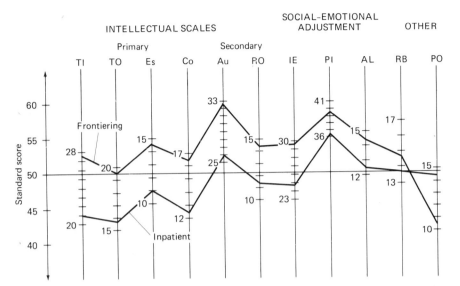

Figure 14-11 Inpatient vs. frontiering. The upper line represents the scores of the frontiering group (the least traditional group). The lower line is the inpatient group (the most traditional group.) These are distinct personality profiles with each best adapted to career needs and aspirations.

distinct, but each may be best adapted to the needs and demands of its own careering aspirations.

Every baccalaureate nursing program, whether designed for the novice or for the educationally mobile, sends its graduates into some facet of professional nursing practice. Breadth and intensity of professional interests, as well as self-reports of competence, although significantly *different* among the five orientation groups, bear no significant relationship to traditionalism. On these measures, the community resembles the in-patient group in scoring lower, whereas the vertical mobility resembles the frontiering and academic groups in their higher scores. Thus, while studies of Second Step students support the notion that the educationally mobile nurse tends toward a nontraditional orientation, let us not lose sight of the fact that many important characteristics are *not* correlated with traditionalism.

No significant differences occur on a measure of general intelligence. All achieve similar grade-point averages, both in their first and final terms. Strong personal motivations, as well as those of a more practical nature, are equally represented among all five orientation groups. Certain aspects of the Second Step curricular model are equally appealing across the board, bringing students into a baccalaureate program to upgrade their professional qualifications. All are equally willing to encounter adversities in the course of their work with patients and clients. Efficacy, or the sense of one's own ability to bring about change, was not significantly correlated with either end of the traditionalism dimension. Perhaps most important, all appear equally committed to the ideals and values of professional nursing, although the way in which they will express and embody that commitment may vary widely.

On the other hand, as shown in Table 14-2, other attributes of incoming students were strongly linked with the nontraditional or frontiering orientation. Negative correlations indicate that it is the *less* traditional groups who tend to score higher on the NLN achievement tests, as well as on a composite measure of intellectuality derived from personality data. When they discuss their reasons for enrolling in a B.S.N. program, these same students are more likely to speak in terms of specific career-related and educational opportunities, as well as in terms of the purely personal and practical considerations that motivate all students. Already as they begin their upper-division studies, a prime motivating factor for many of these nurses is not to move *into* the hospital setting, but to move out of it. Finally, these nontraditionalists manifest a related cluster of social attitudes: political liberalism, concern with sexual politics, and a decidedly critical evaluation of the present health-care system.

Table 14-2   CORRELATES OF TRADITIONALISM IN
NURSING ORIENTATION

	Pearson's r	Significance Level
External measures		
Intellectual disposition categories[a]	−.28	<.000
Community health score[b]	−.25	<.001
Applied natural science score[b]	−.20	<.004
Motivations: qualitative assessment		
Careering goals	−.25	<.000
Educational goals	−.15	<.001
Avoid hospital employment	−.20	<.000
Self-report data from students		
Political liberalism	−.27	<.000
Effect of women's movement on own career	−.28	<.000
Favors major social change in sex roles	−.18	<.000
Favors major change in health care system	−.16	<.001

[a]Omnibus Personality Inventory

[b]National League for Nursing Achievement Tests

EDUCATIONAL MOBILITY
AND FRONTIERING

We began this chapter with a question about the distinctive characteristics of the educationally mobile nurse. To answer that question, we
have looked at five professional nursing orientations that seem to characterize students who enter postlicensure baccalaureate programs in
nursing. But, you will say, if *all* the students that we have been discussing are entering a baccalaureate program designed specifically for
registered nurse students, and if almost as many express a traditional
in-patient orientation (21 percent) as a nontraditional frontiering orientation (28 percent), what is the basis for this assumed linkage between
educational mobility and frontiering? Put most simply, it is because
two rather different kinds of people enter these programs. There are
the mobile *students*, who are essentially moving only from sophomore
to junior status. And then there are the mobile *nurses* who are actually
returning to school, not just being promoted from one grade level to
the next.

One of the early lessons from the NSSP student data set was that a
common assumption about postlicensure nursing students, that they are
all "mature and experienced" learners, is not necessarily true. Its appli-
cability to a given sample of returning-to-school nurse students depends
in large part upon whether they are enrolled in an upper-division nursing program that stands alone on a campus (often called an "upper 2
program"), or one that is affiliated with an associate degree program
offered through the same institution (often called a "2 + 2 program").
NSSP data were collected from three programs of each type. In the
upper 2 programs, mature and experienced students abound. In the
2 + 2 programs, R.N. work experience, as well as other accoutrements
of maturity (not the least of which are spouses, children, and community
responsibilities), were typically in short supply. With that in mind, let
us look once more at the way in which students are categorized in terms
of orientation, this time breaking the total sample down by type of
educational program. See Table 14-3.

Although both are technically "postlicensure" programs, a stark
contrast occurs between students entering a 2 + 2 and those entering an
upper 2 program. At least in terms of this one dimension, the implication is that these programs are attracting and educating vastly different
student clienteles. The inference is, then, that the mature and experienced learner is the one who is more likely to take to the frontiers.

Extending this line of reasoning still further, I would suggest that
it is not merely R.N. status or even an accumulation of nursing experience that is at the heart of the matter. Rather, it is the nature and timing of the decision-making process itself. The prototypical postlicensure
student has qualified as a safe practitioner, has *functioned* successfully

Table 14-3 TRADITIONALISM IN TWO TYPES OF
POSTLICENSURE NURSING PROGRAMS

Traditionalism in Expressed Orientation Toward Nursing Roles	Type of Program	
	2 + 2 (%) (n = 187)	Upper 2 (%) (n = 250)
Low: 1 = frontiering	16.6	36.4 ⎱ 61.2
2 = community	18.2	24.8 ⎰
3 = academic	12.8	16.0
4 = vertical mobility	19.8 ⎱ 52.4	11.2
High: 5 = in-patient	32.6 ⎰	11.6

in that capacity, and has then, at some subsequent point, made a conscious decision to *change directions* and to enroll in a B.S.N. program.

Such a choice is not easy to make. It may require an agonizing reappraisal of former assumptions and priorities; it may entail considerable risks; and whether or not it was the "right" decision may continue to plague the student, especially as the first round of mid-terms rolls into view. Yet this very process of self-appraisal may best define the uniqueness of the educationally mobile nurse, by creating an expectation of self-change and by establishing a readiness to supplant an "old" nursing identity with a new one.

Our research provides no statistical proof that this decision-making process engenders also a readiness to reexamine the traditional boundaries of the nursing profession and to venture onto the frontiers. Yet we have reviewed a compelling array of evidence which points in that direction. Having redirected their own energies and aspirations, these ambassadors between the two "worlds" of nursing may stand ready to extend and expand the meanings of nursing practice.

REFERENCES

Heist, Paul, and George Yonge. *Omnibus Personality Inventory Form F Manual*. New York: Psychological Corporation, 1968.

Jako, Katherine L., and others. *Demonstration Study of a Second Step Nursing Program*. (HRP #0900617). Springfield, Va.: National Technical Information Service, 1978.

——."Frontiering: An Emergent Concept for Nursing Research," in *Proceedings, Vol. 1: Researching Second Step Nursing Education*, ed. Katherine L. Jako (ERIC: ED 194 790). Rohnert Park, Calif.: Sonoma State University, 1980.

——."Five Professional Nursing Orientations," in *Proceedings, Vol. 2.: Researching Second Step Nursing Education*, ed. Katherine L. Jako. Rohnert Park, Calif.: Sonoma State University, 1981.

15

Back to Work: More Transitions?

Donea L. Shane, R.N., M.S.
Joan Dixson, R.N., B.S.N.
Myra Moldenhauer, R.N., B.S.N.

Among the uninvestigated aspects of the nursing educational mobility movement are a series of questions relating to the feelings, attitudes, career paths, and effectiveness of nurses who have successfully returned to school, graduated, and then reentered the nursing workplace with new and additional credentials, knowledge, and skills.

As a means of starting to investigate these questions, we asked two graduates of a B.S.N. nursing program to reflect upon their experiences, feelings, and life changes since graduation the second time. These two individuals were chosen because they were known to be mature, reflective individuals and had been successful students while in school. In addition, they had been out of school long enough to have had time to experience transitions. The results of the rather nebulous charge given to them are the two vignettes that follow. We have no way of knowing if the stories these two writers tell are typical or unique. We present them simply as the honest, straightforward presentations that they are. Here is what two people report about their after-graduation thoughts, feelings, and life changes; inevitably, they reflect upon how the state of the nursing profession has affected their lives and nursing practice.

Joan Dixson is in her thirties, a wife and mother of two, and is currently a head nurse in a rehabilitation unit in a medium-sized urban hospital. Myra Moldenhauer is also in her thirties, unmarried, and the in-service assistant in a postanesthesia recovery room in a typical hospital. Each were successful students during their returned-to-school years. Joan's first nursing education occurred in an associate degree school; Myra first graduated from a diploma school. Each attended the same baccalaureate program, but were in different years and did not know each other. Let's hear Joan's story first.

JOAN'S STORY

I remember when I first became a nurse. That R.N. behind my name was the most important thing I'd ever done for me.

The first staff nurse position I held was on a busy surgical unit. I remember being enchanted and envious of the experienced nurses around me. I also remember labeling a few as frustrated, bitter and cold-hearted.

One year later I found myself orienting a new graduate to the unit, and I heard myself say words that I used to think of as "bitter, cold and frustrating." How I had changed in one year! I didn't know what to call it then, but I later found out I had been through "reality shock."

To make a long story brief, some years later, I found myself back in school, working toward my B.S.N. degree. After several years of frustration, tears, hard work, and occasional laughter, I was a nurse again, only this time I had a degree to add to my credit.

And I lived happily ever after? No, I didn't, to my great surprise. After a very short period of employment had passed, I found myself frustrated, bitter, and perhaps more angry than I had ever been in my life! I had been "had," not once, but *twice* by my chosen profession.

Furious, I turned to teaching nursing at a two-year nursing program. There I was able to talk about what I wanted nursing to be, and to take fresh minds and hands and say, "Watch me and listen! This is the way it should be." I was fighting my own private battle against the gap that I fell through twice. I identified that gap as one between theoretical nursing and clinical practice.

Eventually, I returned to clinical nursing in a hospital setting and worked as a staff nurse for several years. Then I accepted a head nurse position, just about the time I was feeling restless, frustrated, and more or less "dead-ended."

In thinking about my nursing employment I have honestly come to believe that I have given up (or perhaps "copped-out") three times on my profession. And the irony of it all is that I love bedside nursing and I think I'm good at it.

In one more attempt to explain to myself why I am so disappointed in general nursing job satisfaction, I made a list of questions that seemed pertinent to my quest. I quickly answered these questions, put them away for three months, and then looked at them again.

As I reread my personal survey, I realized that I didn't totally agree with my original answers. So I interviewed thirteen other nurses from the Midwest and Southwest who had returned to school and were re-employed in nursing for at least eight months after graduation number two and put the questions to them. My survey is small, but it is their responses I wish to add to mine and share with you.

My first question I wanted answered was "Why do nurses return to school?" Several respondents said they wanted to qualify for better pay by virtue of having more education. Another response was to learn more about the theories of their profession. One nurse said she wanted to hold a more responsible position. She was then quick to clarify this, saying this did not mean additional responsibilities, but working higher up on the ladder of leadership. She felt stressed at the responsibility she already had as a staff nurse. One general response that most nurses acknowledged was in the area of frustration. Most told me that they felt perhaps if they knew more, had more letters behind their name, then maybe they could be happier and "get ahead." "Getting ahead" seems to mean learning the political ways to get out of routine staff nursing but still maintaining a clinical practice within the employment situation, or it means decreasing the amount of pressure felt as they worked in their professional setting.

Burn-out is one major reason nurses return to school according to half of my respondents. The thought behind this is that if you gain more knowledge maybe reality shock won't happen to you.

No one disagreed with the ideas that decreasing pressure in work and decreasing responsibilities to tolerable levels was a big factor in their decision to return to school. Several nurses felt very strongly that some nurses stay in school "forever," just to avoid the pressure, stress, and conflict of daily nursing employment.

If I may draw a subjective conclusion, I would say that reality shock itself might be a prime motivation in nurses seeking advanced nursing education.

Another question I wanted answered was whether nurses feel reality shock when they return to nursing employment the second time. Shocking news: The overwhelming response was yes! More education has *not* helped nurses to cope with the realities of work pressure. Many students are exposed to M. Kramer's *Reality Shock* and then discuss it. Most discussions get off on the differences in educational preparation and how a two-, three-, four-, or five-year nurse will theoretically function in the employment situation. If schools of nursing truly taught one how to handle problematic issues in nursing, for example, the wide difference between theory and clinical practice, the shortage of good nurses, low salaries, tremendous job responsibilities, and poor hours, perhaps those nurses would have a set of coping strategies that would help them after graduation. Some nurses stated that this one change in educational focus could make a significant impact on the nursing shortage

by keeping those nurses working within the profession instead of dropping out within a year or two of employment. Perhaps nurses are naive
in that they keep returning to schools, professors, or books to solve the
employment dilemma. From my small sampling, it would appear that
these entities do not have answers.

I think nurses use educational advancement to soften the shock of
nursing employment because education is primarily all that is available
to them. I think that this idea might be at the very crux of the matter.
Of course returning nurses suffer from reentry shock. The employment
conditions have not changed! The newly acquired theory and knowledge cannot be truly applied in today's workplaces. The constraints of
too little time, large responsibilities, and understaffing leave few chances
to use an enlarged theory base. The basic function of the nurse is the
same. The conclusions I tentatively reach is that more education has
not helped nurses to narrow the gap between theory and practice.

If education does not lessen the reality shock of reemployment,
the next question I asked was "Did your previous work experience serve
as a buffer against reality shock?" The general response to this question
was yes. Previous work experiences did lessen the reality shock of applying knowledge to function. One nurse said that the shock is still
there, but "because I have already felt it once, it is not quite so flatten-
ing the second time." It seems to be more of a feeling of "It's still the
same" or "It hasn't changed," in talking of work responsibilities and
expectations by employers. Several nurses agreed with my personal
reaction to this theme: increased frustration and anger at the sameness
of the work condition. One nurse put it quite well when she said,
"Time is the biggest factor; education doesn't teach you how to manage
time; it teaches you to set priorities and to assess and reassess. I think
those are very important skills to possess, but I need to know when and
how to find the time to do it."

These are the answers to the questions I first asked of myself and
then of others who had returned to work after extending their nursing
education. These conclusions are very subjective and tentative, but I
can say that, of the nurses I interviewed, one thing is clear. Educationally mobile nurses *do* experience a type of reality shock when they
return to employment settings. It may not be as severe as the first time
they started their clinical practice, but it does happen. Nurses seem
angry about this, and they blame the educational institutions for not
better preparing students for the wide difference between theory and
practice.

They blame higher education rather than the employing institutions for this gap. Perhaps this is because most employers do not acknowledge that a need for change in practice is important or even exists.
In favor of nursing education, one has to acknowledge that educational

institutions do admit that reality shock is a real and present occurrence. Nurses look to education to close the gap, since education is the only side that is willing to look at the problem.

It is a large, loud silence that nurses like myself hear when they ask for an answer to "Why is working in nursing so different from what is taught?" There is no one answer to the question. Perhaps we just keep validating the problem.

MYRA'S STORY: THE BACK-TO-WORK SYNDROME

The Bicultural Nurse Graduates and Has a Honeymoon

It was December 14, and Christmas, for which I was totally unprepared, was only two weeks away. However, my concerns about the holidays were overshadowed by an enormous sense of relief. I had finally lived through the last of thirty incredibly stressful months as a full-time B.S.N. student, part-time staff nurse, and sometime human being. Along with my colleague–classmates I had been through most of the stages of the returning-to-school syndrome several times. Nonetheless, I now felt immensely unburdened and euphoric (and therefore truly bicultural).

As a diploma graduate who had seen twelve years of front-line, full-time hospital practice, I had initially been excited about both "moving up the career ladder" and "expanding my knowledge base." Returning to school for my B.S.N. had accomplished the latter. I had read more material than I could possibly absorb, learned some new concepts, and updated some old ones. I had honed, polished, and broadened my philosophy of nursing. I had also wasted a lot of precious time.

There had been many occasions when I had performed what were, to my adult mind, impossible, even ludicrous, gyrations in order to complete the program. But that was now in the past. As one of the graduation speakers, I waxed eloquent on the virtues of baccalaureate nursing education in general and the college of nursing in particular. I had, after all, benefited from my school's special provisions for R.N. students.

Furthermore, the last semester of the program had been a hectic but largely positive experience. In spite of the incredible volume of work required and the redundant tedium of eight hours a week in a critical care rotation, I began to "feel different" about my student role and about nursing in general. I had the great good fortune to have my ICU rotation supervised by a bicultural faculty member who effectively communicated both confidence in my abilities and empathy for my feelings. That this same faculty member was also the senior level coordinator may have contributed to the change in attitude I began to sense in both myself and the faculty. This was especially true of the community health rotation, which was a refreshingly new experience for me.

In community health, I was suddenly free from the pressure to perform the specific tasks often dictated by the rigid priorities inherent in hospital nursing (especially in critical care, which had been my specialty). I was allowed and expected to determine my own priorities, set my own objectives, and organize my own work. I also experienced the unique viewpoint that comes from having an entire family as a client. Initially, this new role had been stressful, but as the last half of the semester rolled around, I began to revel in it. I had had a taste of autonomy during my recent years in nursing administration, but never to this degree and certainly not when it came to planning and delivering nursing care. My self-concept, as reflected from faculty attitudes, was changing from that of "dependent, subordinate student" to "student colleague."

Thus the senior semester ultimately became the most gratifying of all the "substantial nursing content" I had endured. I felt both challenged and supported by the faculty. In meeting that challenge I had pushed myself to new levels of stress and exhaustion, but I had begun to have a vision of what the practice of nursing could be. In a word, I had been "resocialized."

The Bicultural Nurse Encounters Substantial Real-Life Content

Because of my mostly positive senior experience, I approached graduation with fond delusions of grandeur. I envisioned graduate school, perhaps even a doctoral program. I mentally rehearsed history-making speeches to the assembled delegates of ANA and fancied that I might single-handedly heal the breach between nursing service and nursing education. My new B.S.N. was the down-payment on my ticket to fame, fortune, autonomy, and self-actualization. Having "expanded my knowledge base," I was now ready to "move up the career ladder" . . . someday.

First things first, however, and the first thing on the agenda after graduation was a champagne party. After that, I immediately launched into holiday festivities, followed by a long-delayed trip home to see the family. In short, I now had time to be a Real Person.

I would like to digress for a moment to share my concept of Real People. Real People take care of themselves in a more-or-less holistic fashion. They make a living wage and function as full-fledged members of hearth, home, and social group. They do not suffer from acute role conflicts. They do not dance to the tune of incessant stress and chronic fatigue. For the most part, they lead balanced, integrated lives.

As a Real Person, I was more than willing to relegate fame and fortune to my fantasies for the present. On graduation day I had caught a cold that was still going strong in January. I was exhausted, in debt, in need of health care, and certainly in no shape to begin revolutionizing the nursing profession. My personal care plan did not include high-level stress. I needed time to regain equilibrium.

I therefore chose to remain in my current staff nurse position, because the work schedule, salary, and benefits were good, especially now that I could work full-time. I briefly considered other options but could not seem to muster the energy or motivation to really pursue them. I had vague fears of "failure," or making less money, or getting a community health job one year and having funds for it cut the next, or encountering some strange new reality shock, or who knows what?

I had nightmares of eventually returning to hospital work, of "starting all over," working odd shifts and weekends, working my way back up the seniority ladder to the "choice" staff nurse position I now enjoyed. (After all, I already had something any sane hospital nurse would covet: a day-shift job with at least every other weekend off in a reasonably well-staffed unit.) I still occasionally have those nightmares.

On the other hand, I was well aware of the career disadvantages of staying where I was. In my present position, my new B.S.N. was more or less superfluous. There would be no increase in salary or status. The system as a whole would have no new expectations of me. I could coast for awhile if I wanted to. Or could I?

I did not pause to reflect that the above-mentioned fears and attitudes were those of the well-socialized hostpial nurse who was still very much a part of me. Perhaps this was because I had some new attitudes as well. Phrases like "role model," "change agent," and other such sugar plums now danced through my head. If I could not immediately return to academia, perhaps I could incorporate a bit of academia into the work setting.

Overall, it had seemed a pretty good coping strategy to avoid the stress of a major career change. I had heretofore functioned adequately in my part-time job but had reserved most of my emotional and psychic energy for school. It did not occur to me that the focusing of this energy on full-time, real-life hospital nursing would constitute a major transition in and of itself.

The Bicultural Nurse Vacillates and Occasionally Integrates

The upshot of all that postgraduation ambivalence was that I reentered the mainstream of nursing practice with the contradictory goals of functioning on a higher plane while taking it easy for awhile. Having been newly introduced to the joys of nursing research, I had in mind to do a clinical research project such as would have rendered a member of the nursing faculty ecstatic. My co-workers, however, were less than ecstatic, although some agreed it might be a "nice thing to do." When it became apparent that such a project would involve many extra hours of work (and probably politicking), I abandoned the notion.

Still, I felt a need to do "something extra." So I began to ask about the possibility of presenting an in-service course. This, too, required extra work on my own, but it was not a new skill for me. It eventually proved to be a gratifying experience, especially since it allowed me to use and feel rewarded for some of the "nontechnical" skills and concepts that had seemed so important in the academic setting.

Another such experience was my brief service on a unit committee to formulate budgetary justifications for new equipment. Here, writing ability became important.

During both of the above-mentioned "special projects" I noticed a definite upswing in my morale. But what of the day-to-day nursing care that has constituted the bulk of my activities? Is my B.S.N. truly as "superfluous" as it has often seemed? The answer to that question is not an easy one. Postanesthesia recovery care requires a fair amount of technical ability, much of which I already had before I went back to school. However, I have noticed some differences in my nursing approach on both a subjective and objective level.

One slow morning while I was plodding through a "routine" recovery room admission and my mind had a chance to drift a bit, I had one of those "aha!" experiences that can be so much fun. It suddenly reoccurred to me that what I had regarded as "using my head" in relationship to procedures and protocol was none other than *the nursing process*.

This overstatement of the obvious may not seem so strange when one remembers that, with some exceptions, the jargon is different in the grass-roots hospital culture. There nursing is often perceived in terms of tasks to be completed, doing a good job, carrying one's fair share of the load, and other such human issues of survival. As we have seen, it was very easy for me to use and think in terms of such concepts out of long years of habit and something more: the basic need to be part of the group.

At any rate, I no sooner began to remember that this was indeed, "the nursing process" than another light began to flicker. On further reflection, it occurred to me that, whenever our nursing care was not quite as effective as it might have been, the cause could generally be traced to a "short-circuiting" of the nursing process. Usually this meant that our data base had been incomplete and/or our physical assessment less than thorough.

To summarize, then, one difference that my B.S.N. has made is that I am now more conscious of when and how I and my colleagues use (or fail to use) the nursing process. From that point, it has not been difficult to relate to other aspects of nursing in a more conscious and deliberate way. Such concepts include "accountability," of which I need have no fear as long as I am engaged in the *process* for which I am duly educated and licensed, and "documentation," which provides not only "evidence" of the process but a tool to facilitate continuity of care. (I am frequently teased about my voluminous charting.)

Lest the reader be overwhelmed by these earthshaking revelations, let me be quick to say that I don't necessarily spend all my days being euphoric about the nursing process. There are times when I pull back emotionally and wonder, "So what? Who cares, really, just so long as the job gets done?" On that morning when I felt "aha!" I didn't tell anyone. Had I done so, my co-workers would probably have chuckled, shook their heads, and told me to take a break.

My colleagues are like that. They often express amazement, puzzlement, or sometimes out-and-out disapproval toward some of my nursing approaches. Their responses range from a friendly "Slow down, you're making me nervous," and "That's not the way we're supposed to do it," to "Come tell me what you think of this patient." Overall, I think, we have learned from each other.

Comments about my B.S.N are equally varied. There is the joking admonition, "Ask her. She's smart. She went to school." There are also more serious and sincere questions like, "Why don't you apply for that head nurse position?" or "When are you going to *do* something with your education?"

That is a good question. It is now over a year since graduation. The nursing profession remains unrevolutionized, and the assembled delegates of ANA have never even heard of me. I am definitely behind schedule. I am increasingly aware of feeling that personal pride in using the nursing process has its limits toward achieving self-actualization, not to mention some of my other more basic needs. I am also aware of beginning to feel highly selective about the kind or quality of stress I want to deal with in my career. This is why becoming a head nurse (with some exceptions) is not appealing. Furthermore, I find myself weighing the difference in financial and societal rewards granted to those with a graduate education in nursing compared to those with graduate preparation in other fields.

Nursing, it seems to me, has been a "troubled profession" almost since its inception, and greater talents than mine have seemed unable to affect significant, broad-based, grass-roots change. I am beginning to doubt that the gap between education and service will ever be bridged, because that gap is the distance between what could and should be (idealism) and what really is (pragmatism). Like it or not, we live in a capitalistic, materialistic, and therefore pragmatic society. In this society, nursing's progress on its own behalf has been real but painfully slow. In that respect, the new public consciousness of the "nursing shortage" should provide our profession with an unprecedented opportunity to unite and take control of its identity and economic destiny. However, when I look around and see what is actually happening, I have the deepening conviction that it is not just I who am "definitely behind schedule."

SOME THEMES EMERGE; SOME ADVICE IS OFFERED

For the reader who is thinking about returning to school, or who is already enrolled in a higher-level nursing program, there seem to be several pieces of advice that we could give, triggered by the vignettes presented in this chapter.

1.   *Your* degree will not magically change *their* workplace. If you return to a familiar workplace, it will have changed very little, while you may have changed a great deal. The staff nurse role in the workplace may have evolved somewhat during your school years, but it is unlikely that a revolution took place while you were gone. Our advice: don't expect changes to have occurred in the staff nurse role.

2.   As you reenter the workplace, your opportunities will be expanded to include roles other than the staff nurse role. Your degree will open doors and opportunities for you. Whether or not you take advantage of these opportunities is, of course, a very personal decision that will be made after you have considered many ramifications. Our advice: taking on the challenge of a completely new role, when offered, provides you with an opportunity to experience unexplored areas of nursing. Try it.

3.   While you are still in school, make efforts to study the areas of nursing that you know are problematic. Develop an armory of strategies that you personally can use to overcome some of the gaps between reality and excellent nursing practice. There are always opportunities to choose the topics of papers, special projects, areas of investigation for group projects. Utilize these opportunities to investigate areas that you *know* are problem areas in real nursing clinical practice. Thus our advice is to use your knowledge of the realities of nursing clinical practice to guide your choices of areas to study while in school.

4.   Reality shock (Kramer, 1974) evidently occurs each time one reenters the nursing workplace world following a sojourn in academia, but repeat attacks are less demobilizing than the original one. Our

advice: read *Path to Biculturalism* (Kramer and Schmalenberg, 1977) before you reenter the work world.

5.   Each of the transitions we are talking about—from school to work, from work to school, from school to work again—can be seen as a similar process (role shock), which is merely occurring in different settings. Thus educationally mobile nurses have opportunities to become real experts in how to minimize or eliminate role shock. Each role transition can be viewed as an opportunity to hone one's skills in flexibly making role changes. Concentrate on how you, as an individual, handle these transitions, and compare your experiences as you make these transitions so that you are consciously learning how you handle these challenges. Our advice: keep a daily journal that records your observations about the role expectation signals you pick up from people in the environment about your new role; record your own feelings as you grow into the new role; compare your various transition experiences as you live through them so that you can detect the commonalities and improvements *you* as an individual have exhibited as you become an expert in changing roles.

6.   Kramer (1974, p. 87) talks about nurses who "lateral arabesque" into teaching nursing as a means of avoiding the realism versus idealism conflict. Joan describes earlier how she attempted this. It is quite possible that you will be offered the opportunity to teach nursing after you graduate, or perhaps you will vigorously pursue an academic career. Another possibility is that you will be offered the opportunity to assume major responsibilities in a nursing service organization. In either situation, you may be in a key position to lessen the gap between nursing service and nursing education. Do you feel it is necessary to reduce the gap? How would you do it, given your scope of influence? As you return to school, in preparation for taking on more complex and influential positions in nursing, keep in mind that this "gap" will be reduced only as individuals become committed to seeing it reduced. Our advice: start right now to sort out your values about whether nursing service and nursing education are committed to roles that are too dissimilar; if you come to the belief that this gap is harmful to the profession, develop ways in which you, as an individual working in a real-life setting (either academic or service oriented), can work to reduce the gap.

In summary, we can see that transitions inevitably occur as people return to work, even if their official positions do not change. These transitions can be anticipated and planned for. Transitions are not inherently "bad" nor are they necessarily debilitating. Do not fear transitions, because they provide tremendous opportunities for growth and change, both to individuals and to the profession of nursing.

REFERENCES

Kramer, M. *Reality Shock: Why Nurses Leave Nursing*. St. Louis: C. V. Mosby Company, 1974.

——, and C. Schmalenberg. *Path to Biculturalism*. Wakefield, Mass.: Contemporary Publishing, Inc., 1977.

16

The L.P.N.-to-R.N. Transition

Susan Woodard Crawford, Ph.D.

The decision to return to school—to reach for the next rung in the nursing career ladder—brings with it a combination of relatively predictable occurrences and, it should be noted, some surprises. While most L.P.N.-to-R.N. students indicate they are prepared to withstand rigorous academic pressures and even make some adjustments in their personal lives, few are able to foresee their reactions to role change within the nursing profession. Many students express bewilderment and frustration that the role of L.P.N., which they felt they had mastered successfully, does not automatically pave an easy road toward becoming an R.N. In fact, there are some instances in which the role of L.P.N. actually appears detrimental, rather than helpful, to learning.

Experience with a number of L.P.N.s in associate degree nursing (A.D.N.) programs has revealed that most students experience this phenomenon, which may be referred to as "role transition." The effective development of programs for L.P.N. mobilists, as the L.P.N-to-R.N. students are often called, has necessitated early attention to role transition and development of teaching strategies that might reduce the trauma of its passage (Crawford, 1981).

Any conclusions regarding role transition must be drawn from the students themselves, who have, by virtue of submitting themselves to an A.D.N. program, provided the necessary data. It is to them that this chapter is dedicated. May the sharing of their experiences assist future students toward a smoother role transition.

L.P.N. TO A.D.N.: YOU CAN GET THERE FROM HERE

A discussion of role transition for L.P.N. mobilists may be facilitated by a brief description of the types of programs available. The oldest and most "traditional" approach requires that the entire A.D.N. program, usually two academic years in length, be completed. From admission to graduation, the L.P.N. mobilist must meet the same program requirements as the student who has had no previous preparation in nursing (often referred to as a "generic" student). Often the only recognition of the student status as an L.P.N. occurs during the clinical experiences, where the L.P.N.'s higher level of confidence and familiarity with nursing procedures may prompt the nursing instructor to provide more challenging situations, as well as to breathe a sigh of relief at not having to cope with yet another "green" student.

An alteration of this traditional approach offers the L.P.N. mobilist exemption from a portion of nursing credits, resulting in "advanced placement" in the program. These credits may be awarded to the student "for being an L.P.N." in what has been referred to as an automatic or *blanket credit* process. Or, as is becoming increasingly popular, the credits may be earned by successful completion of an assessment process designed to validate knowledge and skills gained through prior education and experience as an L.P.N. In either case, the L.P.N. mobilist must meet the majority of A.D.N. program requirements in essentially the same manner as the generic student.

A third and more contemporary approach to upward mobility for the L.P.N. is offered by separate, specialized programs or *mobility tracks*. The student meeting program admission criteria, which may include such stipulations as current L.P.N. licensure, recent experience as an L.P.N., and successful completion of a minimum number of college credits, may enter a program offering exemption from a significant amount of basic A.D. nursing content. Again, credit for knowledge and skills possessed by the L.P.N. may be granted as blanket credit or validated by a formal assessment process.

While this is not the place to launch into detailed descriptions of different types of L.P.N. mobility tracks, a brief outline of an NLN-accredited accelerated nursing program in the upper Midwest may aid in understanding the progression of L.P.N. to A.D.N. role transition. Subsequent to meeting admission criteria specific for this program, the student undertakes an assessment process to validate prior learning and earn credits for L.P.N. education and experience. The formal nursing coursework, which has been abbreviated to three and one-half quarters, follows a theory and correlated practicum format. The first nursing course is an introductory or transition course, specifically designed to begin bridging the gap between L.P.N. and R.N. roles. Two middle courses concentrate on nursing intervention to support individual adaptation in common, recurring health interferences. The fourth and final course requires a synthesis of previous learnings to promote integration of the A.D.N. role.

Why Role Transition?

Although it might seem that the L.P.N. in an R.N. program would have, across the board, an easier time of it than the non-L.P.N., this is not always the case. While the L.P.N. has had previous exposure to some of the theory presented in the A.D.N. program, and certainly more experience with patient care than the generic student, these advantages do not seem to eliminate all the traumas of role transition. For the student in a separate mobility track, which presents nursing content in an accelerated and condensed manner, the very nature of the program is conducive to a more rapid, and often more stressful, role transition.

Experience with L.P.N. mobilists pursuing a "fast track" to earn the A.D.N. has revealed some predictable patterns in role transition, which have aided us in structuring the program in an attempt to minimize stress and to facilitate integration of the new role. We have observed that the progression of role transition appears to correlate with the layout, or sequencing, of the program. To illustrate, during their initial exposure to information about the program, most students exhibit attitudes ranging from extreme optimism to some hesitancy regarding their ability to succeed in the program. The subsequent assessment process for validation of prior learnings seems to bring students in touch with a more realistic appreciation of what is required to become an R.N. At this time, the possibility of failure looms as a tangible threat. Finally, the nursing coursework itself both precipitates and promotes acquisition of the new A.D.N. role. A more detailed look at student reactions to these phases, and especially how they affect role transition, follows.

EARLY PERSPECTIVES

The fact that most L.P.N.s initially hear about mobility programs from other L.P.N.s, some of whom have survived such a program, can have both positive and negative repercussions. While it has been encouraging to learn that word of our program has traveled along both local and national grapevines, we have found that by the time some of the information reaches potential students it may either be outdated or distorted.

In an attempt to accurately respond to the questions commonly asked about the program, we have prepared a somewhat detailed information letter that describes admission criteria, program requirements and progression, and the application process. Immediately following acceptance into the program, students attend a detailed group orientation where we try to "tell it like it is." This two-hour session, which outlines all aspects of the program and specifically speaks to our expectations of the student, is designed to generate enthusiasm while, at the same time, presenting reality. We have found that a straightforward and informative approach tends to both reassure and encourage those who are highly motivated, while presenting realistic options to the more tentative and ambivalent. In addition to clarifying information regarding the academic aspects of the program, it is our intent to encourage early consideration of some of the more common personal and professional adjustments that may need to be made as students enter and progress through our program (Wooley, 1978). Following this group session, some students may arrange individual conferences to discuss specific needs.

How Do I Feel Now?

In these early stages of role transition, one of the most striking and recurrent sentiments expressed by the L.P.N. mobilists is that such a process will occur without much ado. This "honeymoon" attitude seems to be one of pride and positive expectancy. The students feel they are competent L.P.N.s who have the ability to become R.N.s and are excited about returning to school. They may have some qualms about successfully completing college-level work, but they are confident they can integrate the student role into their other existing personal and professional roles. They can verbalize that "Yes, there will be some adjustments," but, after all, they are adept at coping and are prepared for most of the pitfalls. "Others may find role transition a struggle, but not us!"

A sample of typical comments from incoming students may serve to illustrate some of the feelings experienced by those seeking to change roles. One L.P.N. mobilist who had functioned for several years in an intensive-care unit in a private hospital stated that, when she told her relatives she was "going back to school to get my R.N.," one said, "Oh, then you'll be a *real* nurse." Her reaction was one of anger, as she felt as an L.P.N. she had been a "real" nurse all along. Another student recounted an instance where a patient asked her, "Are you a nurse or an L.P.N.?" Again, there was the implication that the L.P.N. was "less than" a nurse. An attitude expressed by many is that they are currently in responsible positions and are doing the same work as R.N.s. "I'm tired of being treated as the lowest member of the staff. If I'm going to do the same work, then I want the same respect and salary for it!" Some admit that they see their progression through the A.D.N. program as a credentialing process to ensure them payment for skills they already possess and are performing on the job.

A widespread feeling that may be detected among many of our entering students is that they want an accelerated type of nursing program so that they can complete it quickly and take licensure exams, and, concurrently, they want to work full-time as L.P.N.s! A typical statement is "Because I'm a good L.P.N. the program should be easier for me . . . I plan to put myself through with my L.P.N. job." As the students progress through the program, we will see how these initial impressions may become modified.

The Assessment Process: Am I OK?

In our program we employ a dual assessment process: (1) the testing of nursing theory using objective examinations, and (2) the testing of nursing practice in both the on-campus laboratory and area clinical facilities. During the assessment of theory, students have some of their initial enthusiasm restrained by the work and worry that goes into studying for credit by examination. In this phase, which I like to call "honeymoon with reservations," most of the students retain their confidence and optimism but begin to realize that the credentialing process will not be automatic. Some students, already feeling pressures exerted by the multiple roles of student, wage earner, and family member, become defensive and demanding. The fear of failure, of not retaining eligibility to continue in the accelerated nursing program, becomes of concern to many. Already some students are beginning to realize that they will need to reduce their work hours in order to study harder and succeed in the program.

Prior to the testing of theory, which we accomplish through the use of national standardized examinations, some students have been heard to remark, "I'm sure I won't have any trouble passing these tests. I've been an L.P.N. for nine years." Others are less sure. "I think I know the content—after all, I'm a competent L.P.N.—but I'm afraid the test questions will be worded in such a way that I'll miss them."

During the assessment of practice, which follows successful completion of the theory examinations, a more confident attitude prevails. Most students report diligently reviewing the examination study guides, and they appear to approach the testing of their nursing skills in the college laboratory and hospital with a positive outlook. An exception to this is students who have been L.P.N.s in a clinic or long-term care facility and are unsure of their ability to perform some of the procedures required in an acute-care setting. Again, the prevailing attitude at this time seems to be that of pride in being a successful L.P.N. and confidence that this role will make the transition to the new role of R.N. easier.

ROLE TRANSITION IN EARNEST: THE TRANSITION COURSE

Having survived the admission criteria and the assessment process, L.P.N. mobilists begin the three and one-half quarter nursing course sequence with a transition course designed to set the stage for L.P.N.-to-R.N. role change. Presentation of new content addressing the philosophy and framework of our program and expectations of the A.D.N. role is followed by a heavy emphasis on utilization of the nursing process. While this may seem, at first glance, to constitute a review of prior learnings for the L.P.N., it soon becomes apparent that the nursing process, as we present it at the A.D.N. level, differs greatly in depth and scope from what most L.P.N.s are familiar with.

As seems to be the case with nursing mobilists at other positions on the career ladder, our students fall prey to the previously described returning-to-school syndrome or RTSS (Shane, 1980). The initial honeymoon phase of enthusiasm and excitement regarding the return to academia begins to fade about the time that students are pressed into applying their new-found and more complex version of the nursing process to clinical nursing practice. The emergence of the conflict stage of the RTSS brings with it the cold, hard reality that role transition may take some effort, after all.

Why Am I Struggling?

For the majority of students, abandoning the honeymoon stage and experiencing the early stages of conflict comes as a bitter disappointment. Initial experiences utilizing the nursing process, which many students felt they had previously mastered, finds them clinging to their original identity as L.P.N.s—specifically, the way they function successfully as L.P.N.s in their present jobs. When their performance in theory or practicum falls below the level of competence required by the program or expected of themselves, many students voice frustrations and may become defensive. We hear statements like "But I've always done it that way," or "If I had more time, I know I could do better," and "Is all this stuff really necessary to become an R.N.?" It appears that, although the L.P.N. mobilists have taken this step toward a new role, there is inward resistance to internalize that role without a struggle.

Compounding the woes of adjustment to a new nursing role are the multiple effects that returning to school has on already existing roles. Most students, in addition to feeling that they need to solicit moral support from family members, discover early that there must be multiple role changes within the lives of themselves and others in order for them to survive the return to school. Work patterns are disrupted as many L.P.N.s alter their job schedules and even their places of employment to fit the school calendar. Friends, who were initially supportive of the back-to-school endeavor, feel neglected and find it difficult to understand that the student feels compelled to put previously enjoyed activities and relationships in the back seat in order to study. Community responsibilities, including involvement in church, recreational, and child-related activities, are curtailed or even suspended for the duration. In some instances, students commute for long distances or even move to our suburban locale from rural areas in order to attend the program. And, as always, the problem of sufficient funds for tuition as well as living expenses looms as a significant and sometimes underestimated consideration.

In an attempt to minimize these stresses (and in response to comments from students themselves), we have added an admission criterion requiring completion of fifteen college credits before entering the program. Our students, many of whom have never attended college, now have a chance to become adjusted to this new educational environment before having to cope with nursing role transition. In addition, the completion of fifteen college credits reduces the number of remaining credits needed to complete the program, thus lightening the quarterly academic load.

A view from educators in our nursing mobility program reveals that, while students seem confident and proud to have begun the program, many of them present an "overloaded profile"; they are attempting to combine the new student role with that of wage earner (to support themselves and often a family as well) and a multitude of other interpersonal roles. We see a tendency on the part of students to attempt to place their life situation problems, many having to do with health and interpersonal relationships, into the background while they concentrate on the student role. It appears that acquisition of the new student role must effect a change in existing roles or the consequence of role overload is likely. Many of the students need assistance with setting priorities, being appropriately assertive, and managing stress.

An excerpt from the diary of a student nearing completion of a transition course may serve to illustrate the pressures experienced by many at this time.

> I'm in the process of figuring everything out. My roles have changed, and therefore the roles of my husband, son and friends have changed. I was having a lot of trouble trying to go to school and work full-time as a nursing supervisor. This next week is my last week in that position. I decided to work "on call" in four different facilities so that I can pick my hours and days to work based on school and family needs. I really feel good about having made that decision.
>
> Also, I'm enrolling my five-year-old in an all day (6:30 a.m. to 4 p.m.) accredited private kindergarten program. I needed to do something to ease the stress of finding babysitters who would put up with my schedule. Also, I feel that my son needs more consistency. I feel good about this decision also!
>
> Everything is not <u>so</u> positive though. I find myself blaming my schedule with school (etc.) for anything that goes wrong. I need to learn not to do that. I always feel bad when I have those "fleeting thoughts."
>
> I started out thinking the program would come and go without too much problem (as did, I suspect, most people). But I have found that everything you said would happen is happening.
>
> I really enjoy school and I now am starting to realize the difference between an LPN and RN—(I really didn't understand the difference before). I always thought I was a good nurse; it didn't matter if I was an LPN, I was just as good (or better) than an RN. I would be embarrassed if I found out no one else felt this way. Also, I'm finding that the more I learn, the less confident I am that "I know it all." I think all these feelings are a positive factor in the role transition from LPN to RN.

Help!

To help ease the students' passage through the early dark tunnels of role transition, we have developed a learning module that is based on the rationale that the L.P.N. mobilist experiences significant changes in function and position which have implications for personal and professional growth. We feel that the *process* by which these changes or role transitions occur will be influential in determining the type of *outcome*, or A.D.N. graduate. Therefore, it is essential that the nursing student be aware of role transitions and how they might be effectively facilitated. Only when new roles are learned and internalized is there full commitment to them.

The role transition module is divided into two lessons, which attempt to address the two major areas of stress that we have identified in our students: the transitions from nonstudent to student and from L.P.N. to A.D.N.

The *role transition from nonstudent to student* appears to be the first area needing attention. In this first lesson of the role transition module we attempt to assist the student to recognize implications of the move from nonstudent to student, and to effectively utilize both internal and external resources to facilitate this transition. Students are required to examine characteristics of the adult learner as they might pertain to themselves. Many students seem relieved to perceive that they are not alone with regard to these traits. Next, we have them compare this nursing program's philosophy of self-directed learning with the concept of other-directed learning, which most of our L.P.N.s appear to be more familiar with. Finally, students are directed to scrutinize carefully each area of their lives that may be influenced by the new student role and to consider constructive steps for adjusting these roles for compatibility with the new identity as student. This seems to be especially difficult for students who have succumbed to the "super-person syndrome": trying to be all things to all people while carrying a heavy academic and work load. Helping them to let go of some of the extraneous self-inflicted responsibilities is difficult, but essential for productive survival. An initial step that I strongly recommend is for homemakers to orient their children and spouses to the mechanical skills of running the washing machine and cooking dinner.

In addition to presentation of theory, students are required to attend weekly self-awareness or small group sessions. These are designed to promote increased understanding of self and, it is hoped, to improve therapeutic communication with patients. The objective of the lesson on role transition from nonstudent to student is to encourage development of an awareness of the *effects* of this transition on self and others and the *processes* by which the transition might be facilitated. Groups of ten students, assisted by a nursing faculty person as a resource, are encouraged to effectively communicate their feelings about these transitions to the group with the aim of helping both themselves and others. Some suggestions for discussion include the following:

1. Discuss the aspects of your life that have been or that you anticipate might become influenced or altered as a result of your new role as student. Share with the group how you already have or would propose to ease this transition.

2. Discuss your feelings about being an adult learner, with particular emphasis on how you and/or others might facilitate (or hinder) the learning process.

3. The return to school may have pronounced effects on *family* roles. Discuss your feelings about these changes, taking into consideration the following:
   (a) The nature of former roles.

    (b) The requirements of new roles.

    (c) Family member adaptation necessary for role transition.

    (d) Methods utilized by you and other family members to facilitate role transition.

    (e) Coping mechanisms needed to deal with increased tensions, conflicts, and the like, that may result.

4. Discuss your transition from nonstudent to student. Be specific in describing how you and others (including the nursing program students and faculty) might facilitate this role transition.

Another big assist to role transition, as identified by students, is the early development of a cohesive peer group. Participation in small group sessions appears to provide a favorable climate for building supportive relationships between students and also between students and the instructor. Finally, the presence of identified L.P.N. mobilist advocates, in the form of nursing and other instructors or college counselors, has been deemed most effective and supportive.

The *role transition from L.P.N. to A.D.N.*, the second lesson in the role transition module, is presented toward the end of the transition course, at which time the symptoms of role transition seem to be surfacing significantly for most students. Originally this content was offered at the beginning of the quarter and appeared to be of minimal assistance. It seemed that students needed to adjust to the newness of the nursing program, and even identify with some of the discomforts of L.P.N.-to-A.D.N. role transition, before they expressed much interest in the topic.

The rationale for this lesson is based on the fact that all L.P.N. mobilists will undergo a transition from one nursing role to another. The effectiveness of this transition and the ease with which it is achieved will depend upon individual strengths, as well as specific learning opportunities. Therefore, it is essential that the L.P.N.-to-A.D.N. transition constitute a continuous learning process that will result in commitment to a new role. It is the objective of this lesson to have students examine role transition with specific emphasis on how it might be most effectively achieved.

Initial content deals with the returning-to-school syndrome (Shane, 1980), as we have adapted it for the L.P.N. mobilist. Students are expected to discuss the syndrome with regard to its incidence, etiology, and stages. The symptoms of each stage are described along with related treatments and even a prognosis. To promote a realistic picture of the A.D.N. role, students contrast National League for Nursing Competencies for L.P.N.s, A.D.N.s, and B.S.N.s with respect to differences in performance at each level. Our program's statement of competencies for the graduate is compared with R.N. role performance (behaviors) actually observed by the student. Next, the L.P.N. mobilist must list R.N. behaviors that are perceived as vastly different from those of the L.P.N. and that must be learned by them for effective performance of the new role.

To understand better the dynamics of role transition, the *change process* is described (Epstein, 1976), emphasizing the clarification of values as essential to internalization of the new role. Students discuss the creation of *psychological safety* (the reduction of threats or removing barriers to change) as an aid to better learning. At this time, we encourage them to be innovative in suggesting ways in which the program, and especially the faculty, might help with reduction of stress and promotion of safety. Finally, we have students identify and discuss specific areas of role change that most likely will be expected by nursing service when the L.P.N. becomes a practicing R.N.

In an attempt to augment L.P.N.-to-A.D.N. role transition theory (Ambruzze, 1974), small group discussions are held. Again, as with lesson one, the objective is to develop an awareness of the *effects* of this role transition on self and others and the *processes* by which it might be facilitated. Furthermore, the effective communication of feelings about this transition to others is perceived as being potentially helpful to others as well as self. Some suggestions for discussion include the following:

1. Review the RTSS. Make *weekly* notations in your self-awareness diary as to the following:
   (a) *Where* (which stage) you feel you are.
   (b) The *symptoms* you are experiencing at this stage.
   (c) *Strategies* that are helping you in adapting to each stage of role transition.

2. Discuss how you perceive yourself in the role of L.P.N. with regard to individual strengths and areas needing improvement.

3. Describe what you feel are "model behaviors" for an R.N.

4. Discuss how you feel about the concept of psychological safety as described in the change process and how this safety might be promoted by self and others during role transition.

5. Compare and contrast the L.P.N.-to-A.D.N. role transition with the "grieving process."

6. Discuss your feelings about making the transition from L.P.N. to A.D.N. with regard to such areas as nursing skills and functions, leadership responsibilities, peer relationships on the job, working with doctors and supervisors, and returning to your present or former nursing location.

THE CONTINUING SAGA:
THE MIDDLE COURSES

Successful completion of the transition course, which heavily emphasized introduction to the A.D.N. role and use of the nursing process, is
not synonymous with an end to role transition. In the next two, or
middle courses, the focus is on nursing intervention to support adaptation during common, recurring interferences to health. Presentation of
content is structured according to Maslow's hierarchy of needs; for
example, the learning modules deal with nursing intervention during
interferences to the needs for oxygen, nutrition, sexuality, fluid balance,
and so forth. Again, the nursing process provides the framework for application of this theory in clinical practice.

Is There No End to Role Transition?

Having successfully mastered the transition course, many students initially feel they are "home free." They have conquered some of the road-
blocks imposed on them and their significant others by the return to
school and approach the remaining three courses in the program with a
degree of optimism. However, it soon becomes evident that the albatross
of role transition is still hanging around their necks. The continuous
demands imposed on them by learning and applying new nursing content quickly move any students who are still honeymooning into the
conflict stage. The majority, already subjected to frustration and un-
rest, continue to attempt to move from conflict toward some form of
resolution.

At this time we see evidence of both negative and positive student
reactions. On the minus side, many students voice disappointment—and
surprise—that the theoretical content is not more familiar to them and
believe that it is presented too rapidly. (This, we remind them, is probably the primary characteristic of an "accelerated" nursing mobility
program.) Some students show a strong resistance to changing their
nursing practice behaviors; there is a tendency to lament "the way we
used to do it," and to hang onto such priorities as speed and efficiency,
valued highly by many of our L.P.N.s. At this time many students,
stressed by personal and student roles, confess to turning to their
"third world" (working as an L.P.N.), where they *are* successful, for
positive strokes. This, of course, serves to further reinforce L.P.N. role
behaviors and may provide a hindrance to effective role transition.
Emotional reactions such as depression, anger, fatigue, and isolation or
indifference may promote or be promoted by less than adequate academic performance. And as for "scapegoating," some of our students

become masters at this art. They persist in blaming their difficulties on a variety of sources, including the program and the instructors. Finally, the feelings of anger and anxiety, which sometimes reach epidemic proportions following the failure of a classmate, may take some time to dissipate.

Accompanying these program-related stresses are the ongoing burdens inflicted upon those close to the students. While many adjustments are continually being made with regard to roles of family and friends, the fact that the program is half over is not always a consolation. One student, responding to a confrontation by her children regarding the effects that schoolwork was having on family roles, stated, "Look, all I ask is that you give me a year." And her child replied, wistfully, "Mom, do you know how long a year is for a kid?" Another example of a child's reaction to having a parent in school is provided by this essay written by the eleven-year-old daughter of one of our students who was just completing the first of the two middle courses.

> It's the weekend when my dad comes home from one of the worst days he's ever had to work. He comes, lies down, and falls asleep. My mom is over studying by herself for an RN degree. Nobody is to bother her or him. My older brothers are out painting the town with their so-called friends, not even thinking what their little sister might be up to. I didn't want to watch TV with some of the dumb programs they have. No one bothers with me. so I end up in my room after suggesting 20 million things to do with my mom. But no, it's always "I've got to study. Why don't you go to bed?"
>
> Ever since I was 3 and up, my mom and dad have worked, and I wish somehow they could make up 8 years to me. I don't care when or where. It's been so very lonely, like I've been had by my parents, and then they just kind of shove me in a corner like I was some kind of toy and my feelings won't be hurt. Now they just don't understand why I want to be with them so very often.

On the positive side—and I'm delighted to report that there *is* visible progress for many at this time—the symptoms of integration begin to emerge. While some students still express occasional feelings of inadequacy and lack of self-confidence (usually during exam time), we have noted that such anxieties tend to steadily decline with each mastery of competencies required by the program. It is amazing to hear students state, with some degree of enthusiasm, that there *is*, in fact, a real difference between their "former" L.P.N. behaviors and their "new" A.D.N. roles. The differences in scope and depth between the two roles is noticeable, and students say they feel relieved to finally understand the "whys" behind their nursing actions. Furthermore, we hear comments like, "Now while I'm working as an L.P.N. I find myself closely observing the ways that the R.N.s give nursing care. Now that I'm in the

program, I'm better able to see the difference between the two roles."
Others admit that while they are working as L.P.N.s they "pretend" to
be R.N.s and to imitate their behavior so that they can more easily
integrate the new role.

Easing the Middle Transition Phase

Although we—and the students—are encouraged by these occasional
"breakthroughs" in role transition and the escalation of attitudes, we
continue to encourage students to seek ways of learning that are as
enjoyable and stress free as possible. All avenues are explored and promoted as possible support systems: family, friends, peers, former L.P.N.
mobilists, the present L.P.N. job, and new learning experiences in the
classroom and clinical area. As instructors, we try to offer both empathy
and constructive advice. The suggestion to students to "make some time
for yourselves," which initially falls on somewhat deaf ears, is finally
accepted by many who confess that this, although difficult to do, is a
necessity.

THE FINAL TRANSITION: SYNTHESIS

The student who reaches this, the final course in our accelerated nursing program, has successfully met challenges posed by admission criteria, the assessment process, the transition and middle courses, and the
myriad of personal and professional conflicts that have accompanied
these sometimes overwhelming academic demands. In this last course,
students are required to synthesize previous learnings into R.N. role
behaviors as they approach that final transition in the sky: A.D.N. student to graduate nurse. This course, following the philosophy of the
accelerated nursing program, is completed in one-half the time alloted
to students in the two-year program. It requires successful completion
of theory (in the form of case studies) and full-day clinical experiences
emphasizing care of groups of patients.

Looks Like We Made It!

The attitude of the great majority of our students at this time is enthusiastic, as might be expected. Most of them profess to have achieved
"complete integration" of the new role and are enthusiastic about syn-
thesizing their learnings. The very few who appear to be in the stages of
false acceptance or chronic hostility seem to want to "just get it over
with and graduate." All students seem a little surprised to learn that

after they have finally adjusted to the role of A.D.N. student they must immediately undergo yet another transition: from protected student to vulnerable graduate.

One of the learning strategies that we employ to assist students with the transition from A.D.N. student to graduate is to have them write diaries of each clinical experience, recounting both positive and not-so-positive learning experiences and describing their feelings regarding their upcoming role as R.N.s. The following is a composite of typical entries from these diaries, which seems to reflect the way many of the students feel at this time.

> Now that we are at the end of this program—and it hasn't been all roses—I'm both excited and scared to become an RN. I think the ideal nurse is safe, caring, and knows a lot about what patients' needs are. What is especially frightening is all the responsibility that I'll have. As an LPN I could always go to the charge nurse. Now I'll be the one *they* come to. I hope I'll be up to that.

Many of the small group discussions during postclinical conferences carry a variation on the same theme: what it will be like as a graduate. While describing R.N. role behaviors, students make comments like, "Now I can see why being a good L.P.N. doesn't automatically mean you'll succeed as an R.N.," and "Although I don't want to go back to school yet, I'm going to take continuing education courses so that I will keep learning. I can see the value of that." An especially interesting comment concerns fellow L.P.N.s. "Just because I'm going to be an R.N. doesn't make me a better person. I'm going to remember where I came from and not treat L.P.N.s like they are second-class citizens!"

Again, as is true through the program, the interpersonal roles of the L.P.N. mobilist are influenced by the approaching graduation. Many students are already feeling pressures from family and friends to take back the responsibilities they had before becoming students. In anticipation of this "return to normalcy," we often hear students say, "When I'm out of school, I'll finally have some time to myself—I'm planning to see my friends again, spend more time with my family, and start some new hobbies . . . ." Additional new transitions may be on the horizon, but at this time, they seem far away.

REFERENCES

Ambruzze, Roberta A. "Role Change—LPN to ADN," National League for Nursing Workshop, December, 1974.

Crawford, Susan W. "Role Transitions," *Inver Hills–Lakewood Community College Nursing Program Manual*, 1981.

Epstein, Rhoda B. "Theory and Process of Change," National League for Nursing Publication 23-1618 (1976), pp. 1-12.

Shane, Donea L. "The Returning to School Syndrome," in *Teaching Tomorrow's Nurse: A Nurse Educator Reader*, ed. S. K. Mirin. Wakefield, Mass.: Nursing Resources, Inc., 1980.

Wooley, Alma S. "From RN to BSN: Faculty Perceptions," *Nursing Outlook* (February 1978), pp. 106-108.

17

The B.S.N.-to-M.S.N. Transition

Patricia Grant Higgins, R.N., M.S.N.

You have had your baccalaureate degree for awhile and now you have decided to return to school again. This time it's graduate school. You want to work for a master's degree. Is attending graduate school different than your baccalaureate program?

WHY A MASTER'S?

There must be a thousand reasons why nurses want their master's degree. Some may perceive it as a way of getting out of a clinical situation that is no longer a challenge. For others, a master's is the route to power and control; others want to develop a clinical specialty. Some may want the intellectual stimulation, others are ready for career changes into teaching, consulting, or administration. Some may want research preparation for the academic life, others perhaps want the joy of seeing a string of letters after their names. No matter why you are considering a return to school, look at your reasons carefully. You will be faced with the demands of a specialized program, so your motivation for returning to school must be strong.

WHAT IS GRADUATE SCHOOL?

An undergraduate program (leading to a bachelor's degree) is a broad intermeshing of concepts that build upon one another over time. Graduate education is achieved in a much shorter time. Most graduate programs require 35 to 50 credits for completion, in contrast to the baccalaureate, which requires 120 to 140 credits; however, the courses in graduate education are complex and demanding. Requirements can usually be met in a year or two. But there are no turtles in graduate education. The pace is exhausting.

CHARACTERISTICS OF GRADUATE EDUCATION IN NURSING LEADING TO THE MASTER'S DEGREE*

The National League for Nursing (1979) has issued detailed statements on the characteristics of graduate education in nursing leading to the master's degree. The master's program in nursing is offered by an institution of higher education and is built upon a baccalaureate curriculum that has included an upper division major in nursing. It provides students with an opportunity to: (1) acquire advanced knowledge from the sciences and the humanities to support advanced nursing practice and role development; (2) expand their knowledge of nursing theory as a basis for advanced nursing practice; (3) develop expertise in a specialized area of clinical nursing practice; (4) acquire the knowledge and skills related to a specific functional role in nursing; (5) acquire initial competence in conducting research; (6) plan and initiate change in the health-care system and in the practice and delivery of health care; (7) further develop and implement leadership strategies for the betterment of health care; (8) actively engage in collaborative relationships with others for the purpose of improving health care, and (9) acquire a foundation for doctoral study.

The NLN stated that individuals prepared at the master's level in nursing improve nursing and health care through their expert practice and through the advancement of theory in nursing. The concurrent study of appropriate graduate-level cognate courses serves to broaden the students' understanding of relevant knowledge from other disciplines. These courses, combined with the expansion of nursing theory that was acquired at the baccalaureate level, permit students to focus their graduate study on aspects of nursing practice and on a functional role that meets their interests and objectives. This combination of relevant graduate cognate courses and advanced nursing theory provides knowledge for the development of expert nursing practice in specialty areas of the students' choice.

Provision for acquiring specialized knowledge and skills in an area of nursing practice may vary in extent and depth depending upon students' goals of specialization. Those preparing for specialized practice roles may concentrate in a single area and have greater opportunities for practice than students ad-

*National League for Nursing, *Characteristics of Graduate Education in Nursing Leading to a Master's Degree* (New York: The League, 1979). Used with permission.

vancing their nursing knowledge and expertise as a necessary element of the functional roles of teaching or administration. Research and consultation skills are integral to the functional roles of specialist, teacher, or administrator, although preparation in these areas is characteristic of post-master's study in nursing. Areas of clinical study should reflect societal needs for nursing services and be sufficiently broad in scope to enable persons so prepared to serve in a variety of settings and locales. It is recognized that some specialty areas in nursing will require depth of knowledge in a delineated area of practice, while others, such as those concerned with services to diverse populations, families and groups, call for an advanced level of generalized knowledge and practice.

The National League for Nursing has further stated that the relationship between clinical and functional preparation is of critical importance. Although advanced clinical preparation is at the base of master's preparation in nursing, the NLN feels it alone is not enough. Functional preparation at the master's level may focus on such areas as the role of specialist, teacher, or administrator. Such preparation is most effective when it provides opportunity for the student to practice functioning within the role. Such role preparation offers knowledge of: (1) the theory of the role; (2) the usual role expectations; (3) the functional dimensions of the role; (4) role ambiguities and conflicts; and (5) strategies for effective role implementation.

In the master's program, opportunity is provided for the student to build upon previously acquired knowledge of the research process, both in conducting research and in helping others to utilize research findings. The master's student in nursing is expected to be capable of identifying researchable nursing problems. The student may conduct replication or pilot studies, or may synthesize a conceptual framework from a review of the literature to design a circumscribed, original study. Knowledge of data analysis is essential both for the implementation of a study and for the intelligent comprehension of research. Opportunities need to be provided to acquire research skills, which can be accomplished in a variety of ways depending upon individual students' needs and goals.

The graduates of master's programs in nursing apply the concepts of change in contributing to the enhancement of nursing and health services. They are actively involved in initiating change and constructively handling the conflict generated when such change is undertaken.

The leadership strategies developed and implemented for the betterment of health care encompass the range of activities needed to influence both nursing education and nursing practice constructively. Furthermore, these strategies are designed to promote the personal and professional investment of self and to employ professional standards and ethical conduct. The leadership strategies emanate from a broad theoretical base and enable the leader to prescribe, decide, influence, and facilitate changes for nursing and health. The direction and scope of leadership are directly related to one's field of operation and to the public served. The roles of change agent and consumer advocate are also effected through the selection and implementation of a broad range of appropriate strategies.

The interdisciplinary collaborative role of the graduate of a master's program is characterized by initiation and interpretation. Master's prepared nurses utilize newly acquired functional role skills to design, initiate, and assume a leadership role as well as a collaborative role. They take an active part in delineating the goals and standards of the group and in designing the mode and terms of operation. One of the major responsibilities of a master's graduate in nursing is to interpret the role and function of nurses to others.

The learning climate for study at the master's level enables students to experience a collegial relationship with peers in their own and other disciplines. Opportunities to relate with faculty facilitate a partnership in learning that promotes intellectual curiosity and creative inquiry and aids in meeting individualized learning goals.

The master's program in nursing is conceptually organized to flow from the philosophy and objectives of the total program and to guide curricular decision making and selection of learning experiences. Such a conceptual scheme also protects the integrity and consistency of the master's program irrespective of the number and variety of specializations, provides a basis for program evaluation, and insures some common learning experience for all students. Because of the diversity of clinical and functional specialties in master's programs, the behaviors expected of graduates should consist of both the behaviors expected of all master's graduates and the specialized behaviors expected of graduates from particular specialties.

These characteristics were developed by the professional nurse membership of the Council of Baccalaureate and Higher Degree Programs and are an expression of professional accountability to the consumer, both student and client.

PREPARATION FOR GRADUATE SCHOOL

Now that you have decided to pursue a master's degree it is important to find a school that matches your interests and abilities. To do this, you have to find out what's out there. An excellent way to begin is to get a copy of the National League for Nursing publication, "Master's Education in Nursing: Route to Opportunities in Contemporary Nursing." You can obtain this annual publication for 75 cents by writing the National League for Nursing, 10 Columbus Circle, New York, New York 10019. It lists all accredited programs with brief program descriptions, tuition cost, and information on financial aid. The listing is organized by state. "Master's Education in Nursing" lists the clinical and functional areas that each graduate program offers. After locating a place and a school that has the program you would like to pursue, the next step is to write for a catalog. The name and address of the dean is contained in this useful booklet, and your request for information should be addressed to this individual.

Choosing a Master's Degree: M.S.N. versus a Nonnursing Degree

Nurses study nursing, law, business, public health, administration, health education, sociology, a host of diverse subjects. For nursing to grow and develop, we need educated men and women. Take some time to look at your career goals. Will a master's facilitate the development of the career you want? If your goal is to teach nursing, do clinical research, or be a director of nursing or nursing service administrator, a Master of Science in nursing is typically required. Most job descriptions in these fields specifically require the master's degree in nursing. However, other career goals can be met by combining nursing with another degree.

Finding the best graduate school for your needs takes time. The time spent is worth it. The choice of a graduate school is very important. Don't rush blindly!

The Master's Thesis

Graduate schools differ in the extent to which research and a thesis are required. Most schools require a thesis. Some schools have a thesis option: either you do a thesis or you take extra course work and a written comprehensive exam. Some schools do not require a thesis. A thesis is a major research and clinical project that requires you to apply research methodologies, including statistics to a problem.

If you have an ambition to complete a doctoral degree, you should do a master's thesis. Many university departments will not consider an applicant who has not done one. If you are planning a career in nursing education, you should do a thesis. Universities evaluate faculty on their research achievements as well as their teaching abilities. Those faculty who have not had the experience of the thesis are at a disadvantage. Taking research courses without the experience of doing a thesis is like reading about how to take a blood pressure without ever practicing the skill.

Many graduate students find they need more than the minimal length of the program to meet all requirements for graduation, including a thesis. For instance, in one recent class only three students completed requirements in the "advertised" three semesters, while over fifty students stayed another semester to complete their research. If a thesis is in your future, pick a topic that you love and can live with for over a year. Spend some time in the library reviewing the literature on your topic of interest. The topic you choose for your thesis may eventually become an important addition to the nursing literature. There is also a need to replicate research studies, describe clinical phenomena, and explore new thoughts and dimensions. One graduate student expressed her concerns over the difficulty in writing a thesis:

> I had difficulty writing my proposal for my thesis. I felt inadequate and almost incapable of doing this task. I indeed had a mental block towards the process. I convinced myself that it was only a big paper and that I didn't have to make a contribution to the profession with my Master's thesis. I only had to learn the research process.
>
> M.S.N., maternal–newborn specialist

Planning Ahead

Read the graduate school catalog very carefully. Note whether or not the graduate program is NLN accredited. Look at the sections explaining the curriculum, faculty, facilities, financial aid and graduate housing. If you know any graduates of the program, talk with them. Careful planning of your graduate program before you start classes can help make a smooth transition into the student role.

Curriculum   The curriculum should be easy to understand. Identify which courses are required and which are electives. Does the curriculum plan provide for you to take electives? If you plan to go away to school, try to take six hours of these elective courses in a university close to home; most programs will allow you to transfer in six credits. These six credits will decrease your course load and allow additional time for thesis work if you are on a tight time frame and must finish the program by a certain date. The course load is usually heavy, so if you can lighten your load, do it.

Faculty   The faculty-to-student ratio is important. The complex nature of graduate school assignments means that graduate faculty cannot teach large numbers of students. The student assigned to an overloaded faculty member suffers because individual needs cannot be met. One faculty member can reasonably advise six to eight students who are working on thesis requirements.

Look at the faculty's preparation. Is there wide representation in educational preparation, clinical expertise, and research skills by the faculty? Have they graduated from a variety of well-respected universities? Do the faculty hold joint clinical appointments in various health-care agencies, a sign of clinical competence and respect? Does the college employ adjunct faculty who are clinicians? The faculty will profoundly influence your life and your nursing philosophy. Try to find honest answers by discussing your concerns with people knowledgeable about the program.

Facilities Examine both the clinical and support facilities. The clinical areas should be inclusive of all specialty areas and include some nontraditional areas in which graduate students may practice. Diverse experiences allow for students to develop specialized clinical nursing skills. The support facilities should include a well-organized extensive library, computer facilities, and laboratories.

Financial Aid Lack of money is a frequent source of stress to graduate students. When writing to the schools of your interest, inquire about scholarships, traineeships, or fellowships. Ask the school about cost of tuition, fees, books, and health-care coverage. The National League for Nursing also publishes a booklet on grants, loans, scholarships, and fellowships (Publication 41-408, 50¢). The deadline for application for funding is often a year before you are accepted into a program. Apply early.

Other Considerations

1. Do you need a car to go to your clinical areas? To give students wide experiences, clinical agencies may be scattered.
2. Some of your classes may be in the late afternoon or evening. This may increase child-care cost.
3. Some schools require an interview. This is a two-way street, as the interview will allow you to ask questions.

> The schools I applied to did not require an interview. But I had lots of questions to ask. I wrote lengthy letters to Deans of the Graduate Schools. One school responded within a week, the others took two months. My questions were important to me and the school which responded quickly made me feel good about myself and took my questions seriously. This was the school I chose for my graduate work.
>
> From a M.S.N. now teaching in a B.S.N. program

Getting Started in Graduate School

You have chosen the school you want to attend; you apply and you are admitted. Getting your life together is the next important consideration. If you must relocate, do so at least a month before school starts. It takes time to find living quarters. In a college town, inexpensive housing does not stay on the market long. Check bulletin boards at school for information ads; sometimes unusual housing arrangements are available in return for light nursing care.

If you are relocating, you will need to become acquainted with the city, since this will be your home for a year or more. The more comfortable you feel with your environment, the less stress you will experience. Early and adequate preparation can be the key to a successful beginning in the master's program.

WHAT IS IT LIKE TO BE A GRADUATE STUDENT?

Study, study, study? This is only part of the total picture. Classes are small with few lectures and many group discussions. Because of the diverse backgrounds of graduate students, conflicting data and opinions make for wonderful discussions. Students lead many classes and discussions, while instructors act as facilitators and resource persons. Activities include writing and presenting papers, meeting various objectives, preparing abstracts and case presentations, conducting research, and much more. Exams, both written and oral, will be required. Creativity is important; there will be opportunities to design and implement programs, develop audiovisual programs, or perhaps develop your own philosophy and theory of nursing.

Some graduate students proceed to the master's program immediately after finishing a baccalaureate program. Others return after being away from nursing for childbearing and childrearing. Many graduate students are experienced in a clinical specialty, while others are interested in making a specialty change.

One graduate student expressed her rationale for returning to school. This comment shows the dilemma that some nurses feel when returning to graduate school:

> I wanted a change. I felt that I needed an additional area of clinical expertise. I thought that by adding maternal-newborn theory and practice to my skills, more job options would be open to me. So I began preparing my family for graduate school two years before I started. I left my husband and three teenage children to attend graduate school in another state. I wanted to come back and teach at the baccalaureate program that I graduated from. Since I don't believe in inbreeding (where a school hires its own graduates as faculty members) I needed to go away to school to pursue my career goals. I was frightened! I went to my new environment a week before school started. I barely found an apartment, got lost on campus, and cried a lot. I knew no one and the phone never rang. For the first time in years, I was responsible for only myself, but I had difficulty adjusting to the quiet which I had always longed for. I now had a room of my own, and it was like a tomb. I really wasn't sure if I had made the right decision. If I couldn't read the map to get around the campus, how could I ever get through graduate school?

> M.S.N., instructor in a baccalaureate nursing program.

GRADUATE SCHOOL RTSS

It is likely that you will experience the role transitions of RTSS when you return to school for a master's degree. Once again, your nursing role will be different and your assumptions about nursing will be challenged.

Honeymoon Stage

A honeymoon period of anticipation and excitement when returning to graduate school is a frequently observed phenomenon in graduate school students.

> There was a refreshing excitement about learning new things and having the freedom to seek answers to my own questions and study in areas of interest. I was enthusiastic about the new experience and happy to escape the staff nursing role which felt so confining at the time.
>
> From a pediatric M.S.N.

> Walking up the steps to orientation, I experienced a moment of overwhelming joy. I was about to be a graduate student. I was special.
>
> From a maternal–newborn M.S.N. teaching in a baccalaureate program.

Conflict Stage

As in the undergraduate RTSS described in Part II, graduate students also experience periods of stress, anger, and hostility. The work and courses are challenging, stimulating, frustrating, and demanding. There is little time for personal pleasures. Questions about the wisdom of one's decision and the worth of the program surface frequently.

Master's prepared nurses were asked to share their feelings about their return to school. Here are some of their comments:

> I felt less competent than I would have expected. Although I'd been in nursing education, the transition back to student life was difficult. I wanted to be directed rather than independent. Looking back, I think part of this feeling came about after realizing that the degree requirements would leave almost no time left for me to explore in depth, 3 or 4 areas of special interest. Disillusioned, it seems that I took the easiest, fastest way out . . . the biggest hassle was learning to "write" after being away from it for nine years.
>
> From a maternal–newborn M.S.N. who teaches in an A.D.N. program.

> Graduate school left me feeling totally lost as to what was expected. I was overwhelmed with the course requirements and everything that would be

needed to obtain an MSN. Having to learn new faces and a new system was probably less threatening to me than to other students in that the school was in my hometown. Also, it was easier for me to get into the swing-of-things having been out of school for only four years.

> From a medical–surgical M.S.N. who
> works in an ICU and plans to pursue a Ph.D.

It was a very stressful time. There were several times I lost sight of all my reasons for attending graduate school.

> From a medical–surgical M.S.N. who is working as an oncology specialist.

At times I felt like I was not treated as much like an adult student as I could have been and many times the hours in the day for work, school, and personal life seemed inadequate.

> From a M.S.N. who worked full-time and pursued an administrator track.

The feelings were mixed, so I felt overwhelmed yet challenged. I also felt frustrated because I wasn't sure the change would be positive. During the first semester, I wasn't convinced the program would make me a better nurse. I now know that it has made a difference. Now the challenge is to convince other nurses that education does make the difference.

> From a M.S.N. who is working as a medical–surgical clinical specialist.

Obviously, students in graduate school experience feelings similar to the conflict stage, but perhaps these feelings are not as dramatically displayed as in the RTSS experienced by undergraduate students. Most programs allow graduate students to plan and write their own goals and objectives. This allows the students direction and control over their course of studies. Also, faculty are usually most willing to listen to students. Both of these dimensions decrease the feelings that nurses have as part of the conflict stage.

> I loved graduate school, it was a great experience. Graduate teachers were more human—they treated students as adults and gave us a "little part" of themselves.

> From a maternal–newborn M.S.N. teaching at a B.S.N. program.

Resolution of Graduate School RTSS

Graduate school could be characterized as a bicultural society. When nurses attend graduate school, they bring with them their clinical knowledge, work experiences, life experience, and an openness to learn. Nurses as students have good feelings about themselves and about the program.

Most students feel self-confident and are there to grow personally and professionally.

> Is this going to be worth it? The answer—yes. Even if you're apt not to change what you're doing already. What you learn and gain personally gives satisfaction.
>
> From an R.N. supervisor with a master's in public administration.

> I gained a lot more in the way of self-confidence from graduate school. Undergraduate school was almost a "tearing down" of self-esteem and graduate school seemed like a "building up" of self-esteem.
>
> From a maternal–child clinical specialist.

Survival Strategies

As we have shown, graduate school RTSS exists. The methods of coping with graduate school RTSS are similar to those described earlier. Self-knowledge—analyzing your typical coping style—will help you to plan strategies that will help you successfully complete the master's program.

As in the undergraduate program, peer-group support is vitally important in the master's program. The group process allows for active listening with opportunities for the expression of true concern for group members. Very often the open communication inherent in the group process helps students accept the reality of the situation and allows exploration of new ways of coping with problems. The group is an active social system, and it can be a major part of your social life while in graduate school. Students quickly learn to divide reading assignments, photocopy summaries of readings, critique each other's papers, study together, and share the ups and downs of life in graduate school.

> I did a lot of group work in graduate school. I loved that sharing of information and experience. It was a valuable part of learning. I got to know some great people and made some long-term friendships.
>
> From a maternal–child M.S.N.

Graduate school RTSS will probably be lessened if you attend the school you received your undergraduate degree from (if you are not concerned about inbreeding). Or it may be lessened if you attend a graduate school in the same geographical area in which you have been living: This reduces the number of role changes you will be forced to make as you enter graduate school. If you have previously attended a small school, you will probably feel more comfortable in a small graduate school; similarly, if you are accustomed to a large, boisterous, complex campus, you will probably be happiest in a large graduate school.

Planning ahead carefully can reduce much of the stress of the graduate program. Utilize your faculty advisor to plan the details of your program. Have a fairly good idea of what courses you will be taking each semester, how you will finance school and your living expenses each semester, how you will schedule work time, study time, and (maybe most importantly) a little time for relaxation and play.

POSTGRADUATE ROLE EXPECTATIONS AND EXPERIENCES OF GRADUATE STUDENTS

After You Finish

How will it feel to have a master's degree? How will other people treat you? When asked this question, nurses responded with the following comments:

> The feeling experienced most frequently regarding my Master's Degree is one of pride. There are times when I feel intimidated, such as the first faculty meeting at the State College where I began teaching. The feeling of intimidation arises out of all the new job opportunities that the advanced degree offers. Challenging jobs of a wide variety are open to the nurse with a master's degree. I experience a feeling of excitement in rising to the challenge of my new job and new role. Intimidation is only one small portion of my post-degree feelings.
>
> From a pediatric M.S.N. teaching in California.

> In fact, I'm smarter, more reality based, and work harder than many PhD's I know. I hope continued education does not reduce my ability to THINK while I learn to conceptualize.
>
> From a maternal–child M.S.N. teaching in Arizona.

> I believe others expect me to know much more than I think I know. Maybe I expect too much of myself and should realize that it will take time, but I feel that I still have much to learn and should remember more than I have from the program.
>
> From a medical–surgical M.S.N. working in Ohio.

Graduate education provides the nurse with the skills needed to do research. It presumably prepares nurses with a knowledge base of where to seek support and information that will facilitate completion of the research. But do nurses feel prepared to do research? Nurses who graduated with their master's were asked, "Do you feel insecure about research?" Here are some excerpts from their comments:

> Somewhat. I question my ability to execute valid and reliable research. The statistics and extraneous variables are difficult components. The nursing role includes the execution of sound research. Research will validate nursing as a science.
>
> From a medical–surgical M.S.N. working as a staff nurse.

> Research, or rather the preparation for it, can be so tedious. I know I can do it, but as a faculty member, I don't have the time. The joke's on me. I have difficulty seeing "so what" research as part of the nursing role. There are so many areas in which nurses need information on which to base their practice.
>
> From a maternal–child M.S.N. teaching at a B.S.N. program.

> Definitely, I do not feel graduate school gave enough practical application in the basics. It was very much "pie in the sky." However, I'm not sure what was realistic to expect in a 12-month program with several areas of concentrated study. Research should be incorporated into daily activities of clinical nursing teaching. To involve more nurses, though, it must be presented in a simpler less overwhelming term. I understand that at graduate level, one must focus on theoretical and statistical concepts, but as a nurse in the "real world," I must be able to develop research projects without the assistance of computers.
>
> From a maternal–newborn M.S.N. teaching nursing in an A.D. program.

> Research has a part in the nursing role. I am still insecure about doing research . . . there are many things that nurses do just because they have always been done that way, but there is often nothing proven about many of these practices. It is very important that nurses do research so as to give evidence that the procedures or practices are either valid or not. It is also important to do research with new ideas which may prove to be more beneficial to nursing.
>
> From a medical–surgical M.S.N.

SUMMARY

Nurses returning to school to pursue a master's in nursing seem to experience the role transitions described in the returning-to-school syndrome (Shane, 1980). The strategies for coping with these transitions include (1) careful planning, (2) use of peer-group support, and (3) choosing an appropriate and high-quality graduate school. Because the thesis is such a prominent part of master's level education, it becomes a focus for much of the anxiety and stress felt during the program. Even after students have successfully completed a thesis, it is possible that they will continue to feel uncomfortable about continuing to do nursing research independently after their graduation.

REFERENCES

National League for Nursing. *Characteristics of Graduate Education in Nursing Leading to the Master's Degree*. New York: The League, 1979.

Shane, Donea L. "The Returning to School Syndrome," in *Teaching Tomorrow's Nurses: A Nurse Educator Reader*, ed. S. K. Mirin. Wakefield, Mass.: Nursing Resources, Inc., 1980.

18

The Master's to Doctoral Transition

William L. Holzemer, Ph.D.
Linda A. Kelly, R.N., M.S.

Returning to school at the doctoral level is an exciting but disruptive process. It influences your personal and professional roles, finances, and ways of thinking. You can anticipate a change in yourself, with a new way of conceptualizing your professional orientation. The selection process requires careful investigation and introspection. This chapter reviews various categories of decisions that must be made in order to select the type of degree, university, and city and to decide whether to earn the degree in nursing or another academic discipline. The pros and cons of these decisions require careful attention to maximize your investment of time and energy in a doctoral program.

It may be helpful to begin this process by reviewing your rationale for pursuing the doctorate. Why do you want to earn a doctoral degree? What is your motivation? The desire to pursue an academic career of teaching, research, and service is the most common rationale. Another significant factor is the desire to move to a top-level administrative position with authority to make decisions that will affect patient care. Increased earning power may also be a motivating factor to earn a doctorate. To fulfill these aspirations, new skills, thought processes, and visions are demanded. Understanding the major reason one has for earning the doctorate will help to balance the competing aspects of each decision that must be made.

The decision to pursue a doctoral degree is a complicated one, and part of this complexity involves the professional and personal goals of the nurse. Individuals considering doctoral study should recognize that doctoral training can serve several professional roles. Education at the doctoral level develops nurses who can evolve theories, conduct systematic inquiry, and teach and administrate programs of nursing care. Most often, however, the doctoral student is required to choose and focus on one of these roles over the others. Despite the differences in professional roles, the purpose of graduate education is to develop nursing leaders who can influence the practice and study of nursing.

Should one pursue a degree in nursing or another discipline? An important article by Donaldson and Crowley (1978) discusses nursing as a discipline, a science, and a practice profession. Nursing as a discipline embodies nursing as an academic discipline, similar to psychology or biochemistry, within graduate education at the major universities in the United States. It has the various trappings or characteristics of a discipline, with a body of published research, research journals, and scientific meetings. The discipline of nursing is becoming well established at major universities in this country.

Donaldson and Crowley (1978) discuss the science of nursing as the knowledge base from which the discipline will ultimately draw its information for teaching and the practice and profession will draw its data for patient care. The science of nursing needs to be further developed. Should you pursue an advanced degree in the discipline of nursing, your responsibility as a new scholar will be to build this science of nursing and to contribute to the growing knowledge base. Finally, Donaldson and Crowley discuss the practice of nursing and the nurturance of nursing. The knowledge base developed by the science of nursing has and will continue to contribute to the improvement of the practice of nursing.

Doctoral programs for nurses in nursing are increasing in availability, although modestly, just as nursing's need for a theoretically based discipline has increased. Preparation at this level would seem critical to the continued development of nursing as a profession, worthy of respect in both the academic and scientific communities (Downs, 1978).

An early statement on doctoral education for nurses was offered by the National League for Nursing in 1955. In the same year the Department of Health, Education, and Welfare's Division of Nursing activated the predoctoral and postdoctoral Nursing Research Fellowship Program to assist nurses to qualify for doctoral study in a discipline outside nursing, to qualify for doctoral study in nursing, and to encourage the preparation of research personnel (Kelly, 1962). In 1955, the NLN offered three assumptions believed to apply to the doctoral degree:

1. The doctorate should not be a third professional degree in nursing but should be based upon a second professional degree and constitute new and enlarged experiences in relevant intellectual

disciplines and scholarly research in the application of such disciplines in nursing.

2. The degree should be interdisciplinary, possibly in the social sciences or education.

3. In those institutions not permitting interdisciplinary doctorals, the degree should be awarded in a single discipline such as sociology or biology.

Prior to 1970, there were only five doctoral programs in nursing. It is understandable why the League was then urging prospective students to pursue graduate education in the social and biological sciences. By the early 1970s the League offered additional principles to guide doctoral education in nursing (NLN, 1973):

1. The doctoral program should be pursued in an established discipline such as the natural, biological, or behavioral sciences with or without a minor in nursing.

2. A program culminating in a Ph.D. with a major in nursing should give candidates a theoretical base in pure research in nursing.

3. Programs leading to a professional degree, e.g., D.N.Sc., should prepare the graduate for the scholarly practice of nursing as a clinical specialist or nurse therapist.

4. Doctoral programs in health care administration, public health, and education should be open to nurses who wish to prepare for such relevant fields of practice.

This statement suggests that there are consistent conceptual differences between the D.N.S. and Ph.D. degree. This assumption is discussed later in this chapter.

In considering a return to school, it will be difficult to decide whether to pursue the degree in the discipline of nursing or in another discipline. There are two levels at which this decision will be made. The first is the practical, pragmatic level and the second is the substantitive level. The practical, pragmatic level suggests that if you are bound geographically to a community that has a university but not a nursing doctoral degree and you choose to return to school, your decision will probably favor a degree in another discipline. On the other hand, if you are mobile, there are exciting programs in nursing available in many states and you will have to choose among them. If you are qualified to pursue doctoral education at one institution, you are probably qualified at others and, hence, you may be accepted at more than one program. However, be sure to apply to several programs as the competition is so keen at some schools that even highly qualified applicants are rejected.

There is growing bias that nurse leaders ought to be focusing their advanced preparation in nursing, rather than in the fields that have traditionally attracted nurses, such as education, psychology, sociology, and anthropology. Part of the reason for this is based on the need for the development of the theory that will guide the science of nursing. Theory development will continue to occur within the discipline of nursing. There is, however, a need for nurses to pursue advanced preparation in social sciences and a great need for advanced preparation among nurses in the basic and biological sciences. Therefore, if your interest is in physiology or chemistry, there is tremendous opportunity to return to nursing upon completion of that program and to become an active leader contributing to the discipline and science of nursing. The expansion of doctoral programs in nursing has increased the options available to nurses seeking doctoral education. Contributions evolving from scholarly work in these other disciplines are highly valued by some leaders in the nursing profession. It is anticipated, however, that the primary development of nursing science will occur within the discipline of nursing.

There are basically three types of doctoral degrees offered in nursing that are post-master's preparation. These include the Ph.D., the D.N.S. or D.N.Sc., and the Ed.D.—the Doctor of Philosophy, the Doctor of Nursing Science, and the Doctor of Education. Table 18-1 presents the universities, the cities, and the types of degrees offered at these respective institutions. There is both clarity and confusion as to the differences among these three degrees. Perhaps the clearest is the Ed.D. offered by only one institution, Teachers College, Columbia University. The Ed.D. is a doctorate of education in nursing. The following discussion is focused on the purported and observed differences between Ph.D. and D.N.S. degrees.

The Doctor of Philosophy is viewed as the most traditional doctoral degree in academia. Those who pursue the Ph.D. are expected to be researchers, to develop sufficient skills combined with a cognitive base to allow them to build the science of their respective discipline. In nursing, the cognitive base is nursing. The D.N.S. degree is viewed by some to prepare advanced clinicians with research skills. The focus on D.N.S. in some of the programs is advanced clinical preparation beyond the master's degree level. However, a recent paper by Holzemer (1981) suggests that there are as many issues of variability within the Ph.D. programs and within the D.N.S. programs as there are between these two types of programs. A prospective doctoral student is urged to explore carefully the particular programs of interest. The type of degree offered is a definite consideration, but it is more important to review the quality of the prospective schools regardless of the type of degree offered. Based upon Table 18-1, the trend suggests that the Ph.D. is the most popular degree.

Table 18-1 DOCTORAL PROGRAMS IN NURSING, 1980 to 1981[a]

University	City, State	Degree offered
University of Alabama in Birmingham	Birmingham, Alabama	D.N.S.
University of Arizona	Tucson, Arizona	Ph.D.
University of California School of Nursing	San Francisco, California	D.N.S.
University of Colorado Medical Center	Denver, Colorado	Ph.D.
Catholic University of America	Washington, D.C.	D.N.Sc.
Rush University	Chicago, Illinois	D.N.Sc.
University of Illinois at the Medical Center	Chicago, Illinois	Ph.D.
Indiana University School of Nursing	Indianapolis, Indiana	D.N.S.
University of Maryland School of Nursing	Baltimore, Maryland	Ph.D.
Boston University	Boston, Massachusetts	D.N.S.
University of Michigan	Ann Arbor, Michigan	Ph.D.
Wayne State University	Detroit, Michigan	Ph.D.
New York University	New York, New York	Ph.D.
Teachers College Columbia University	New York, New York	Ed.D.
University of Rochester School of Nursing	Rochester, New York	Ph.D.
Case Western Reserve University	Cleveland, Ohio	Ph.D.
University of Pennsylvania	Philadelphia, Pennsylvania	D.N.Sc.
University of Pittsburgh	Pittsburgh, Pennsylvania	Ph.D.
Texas Woman's University	Denton, Texas	Ph.D.
University of Texas in Austin	Austin, Texas	Ph.D.
University of Utah	Salt Lake City, Utah	Ph.D.
University of Washington	Seattle, Washington	Ph.D.

[a]National League for Nursing, 1980.

One excellent way to select a doctoral program is to identify a faculty member with whom you would like to study. It is not difficult to locate a mentor prior to admission. After defining an area of interest and locating a major health science university library, start reading.

Discover articles that are exciting to you and then find out where the authors are employed. Faculty are transient and move around, so one has to be careful and not assume that an article published two years ago will correctly identify the school of origin of that faculty member. You can also reverse this process by reviewing recent school bulletins, which list faculty, and then searching the literature for the work of these faculty.

Your academic goals may be unique, crossing traditionally distinct areas such as mental health in an acute-care setting. With this type of goal, you may wish to locate a program sufficiently flexible to allow you the opportunity to design your own academic program.

One question a master's prepared nurse will consider when selecting a doctoral program is whether or not to take the doctorate at the same university that granted the master's. A primary consideration in this choice should be the quality or excellence of the doctoral program. Some institutions may have a strong master's program but a less than excellent doctoral program. All quality factors being equal, the primary advantage of obtaining a doctoral degree at the master's granting university may be continuity. The doctoral degree could be an extension, not a beginning, and there would be continuity with the same professors. However, nursing master's degrees are often viewed as advanced clinical preparation and somewhat unrelated to a school's doctoral program.

If you are a baccalaureate graduate with the career goal to pursue the doctorate, you may wish to inquire if the nursing doctorate program has a master's bypass option. These plans vary greatly at each institution, but it may be possible to enter the doctoral program directly from the bachelor's degree at a few schools.

It is generally inadvisable to earn your doctoral degree where you would like to be employed. If there is a city where you think you would like to live, go to some other part of the country to earn your degree. Become a nurse scholar first and then apply to the faculty with whom you would like to identify and join as a colleague. Many universities prefer not to hire their own graduates because of the danger of "inbreeding." Nurses who have completed a doctorate and who are presented with the possibility of seeking employment where the doctoral degree was earned should thoroughly investigate university policies on hiring and continuing appointment of their own graduates. Furthermore, some doctoral recipients find it difficult to work in the same institution where they have earned their degree because they believe they will always be perceived as a student in the eyes of their former professors, now become co-workers.

To assist nurses considering graduate study, the Consortium Approach to Enhance Graduate Education in Nursing (COGEN) (Curran and others, 1981) was funded by the Department of Health and Human

Resources, Division of Nursing. The primary purpose of this project was to assist nurses in obtaining graduate education. The consortium developed workshops addressing issues to be considered and provided guidelines for selecting a doctoral program. In identifying the potential population of doctoral students, areas of interest and problems they expected to encounter, the project found that a major problem concerned family and personal responsibilities. In addition, doctoral nursing students experienced difficulty with mobility, job security, finances and their roles as spouse and parent (Curran and others, 1981).

For many nurses their present positions provide an essential income with necessary insurance benefits. Giving up either salary or benefits may not be possible. As there are only twenty-two programs for a doctorate in nursing available at present, the potential geographical relocation may create a problem and therefore the factor of program proximity can strongly influence the nurse's selection of a discipline: education, nursing, social or biological sciences. When relocation is not an option, and there is no nursing program available, the nurse should seek doctoral education in a discipline that is available and of interest to the nurse.

Curran and others (1981) suggest that once a program type has been selected, assessment of individual programs should focus on five major questions:

1. What is the overall quality of the school and faculty?
2. What is the nature of the research program?
3. Will graduation from this program enable attainment of personal and professional goals?
4. Is admission into the program a realistic possibility for you?
5. Does personal experience indicate that a student will fare well in this program's milieu?

Other factors to be considered would certainly include:

1. Geographical proximity
2. Availability of financial support
3. Length of program
   (a) Number of credits required
   (b) Duration of residency requirements
   (c) Flexibility of program
   (d) Dissertation requirements
4. Reputation of the institution and program in the profession
5. Current roles of program graduates

Doctoral preparation requires the student to participate in rigorous training, critical thinking, and devotion to a professional life of scholarship. The student in such a program will be exposed to coursework that has not previously been a part of the nurse's practice. The nursing student at this level can anticipate the dilemmas that usually accompany role change. Curran and others (1981, p. 13) suggest that "a careful exploration before making the commitment to candidacy in a particular program and an awareness of the potential academic and personal requirements can reduce frustration and facilitate successful completion of the program."

A frequently asked question from nurses is, "How far does the doctoral degree remove one from patient care?" Patient care has been traditionally understood as the "hands on," direct treatment of a patient's response to physiological or psychological stress. Predicting patient response and developing new options for response and treatment stem in part from clinical experience, but primarily from scientific inquiry. The nurse with the doctoral degree is frequently a practitioner who has added to that role training as a scientist. As Curran and others (1981, p. 13) argue, "If the nurse's future plans include a career focused on research in clinical nursing or nursing theory, educational administration, or that of a basic scientist, then a doctoral degree is essential." Every doctoral student has the ability to determine the extent to which earning the doctoral degree removes her from clinical practice. There is great demand in the profession for the doctorally prepared clinician.

In summary, nurses considering pursuit of the doctoral degree face more dilemmas than the choice of program or type of degree. A major consideration in making the choice is weighing the employment opportunities such a degree offers. Requirements for faculty appointment in institutions of higher education offering a graduate degree seem to be a major factor for nurses seeking doctoral preparation. Nursing faculties in such institutions are expected to meet the same criteria as faculties in other disciplines, and this most often entails having completed a doctorate. Administration of patient-care facilities and services frequently demands a doctoral degree. The nurse participating in policy making is expected to be able to conduct research and suggest innovative methods of implementing health-care services. As the need for an organized body of scientific knowledge in nursing has increased, so has the need for research and evaluation of nursing practice. Peplau (1966) wrote that doctoral education "keeps an open path for highly intelligent undergraduate nursing students for whom the glamour of beginning practice will fade more readily, primarily because of so many unanswered questions." The nurse scholar has the research skills to challenge these unanswered questions.

The returning-to-school syndrome presented by Shane (1980) is a syndrome that is observed even at the doctoral level of education. One sees the conflict stage of being unsure and feeling threatened by the new skills that are demanded of a doctoral student. The bicultural doctoral student is probably the person who can move comfortably and competently from clinician to researcher. Doctoral students seem to achieve the resolution stage sometime during the second or third year.

The discipline of nursing in higher education is preparing a new cadre of leaders with the skills, knowledge base, energy, and creativity to develop the science of nursing. It is an exciting and challenging time to consider returning to school to pursue the doctoral degree.

REFERENCES

Curran, C., M. C. Habeeb, and E. C. Sobol. "Selecting a Doctoral Program for a Career in Nursing," *Nurse Educator*, 6, no. 1 (January–February 1981), pp. 12–15.

Donaldson, S., and D. Crowley. "The Discipline of Nursing," *Nursing Outlook*, 26, no. 1 (1978), pp. 113–120.

Downs, F. S. "Doctoral Education in Nursing: Future Directions," *Nursing Outlook*, 26, no. 1 (1978), pp. 56–61.

Holzemer, W. L. "Doctoral Education in Nursing: Ph.D. or D.N.S.?" Paper presented at Annual Meeting of American Educational Research Conference, Los Angeles, 1981.

Kelly, L. Y. *Dimensions of Professional Nursing*, 3rd ed. New York: Macmillan, Inc., 1962.

National League for Nursing, Council of Baccalaureate and Higher Degree Programs. "Memo to Members." New York: The League, 1973.

———. *Doctoral Programs in Nursing, 1979–1980*. NLN Publication 15-1448. New York: The League, 1980.

Peplau, H. E. "Nursing's Two Routes to Doctoral Degrees," *Nursing Forum*, 5, no. 21 (1966), pp. 57–67.

Shane, D. L. "The Returning to School Syndrome," *Nursing 80* (June 1980), pp. 86–88.

Recommended Reading

In addition to Curran and others (1981), Donaldson and Crowley (1978), and Downs (1978) in the preceding references, the following are recommended:

Crowley, D. "Why Doctoral Education for Nurses?" in *Current Issues Affecting Nursing as a Part of Higher Education*. Papers presented at the 15th Conference of the Council of Baccalaureate and Higher Degree Programs. Houston, Texas, March 1976. NLN Publication 15-1639. New York: National League for Nursing, 1976.

Gortner, S. R. "Nursing Science in Transition," *Nursing Research*, 29, no. 3 (May–June 1980), pp. 180–184.

Johnson, J. E., K. T. Kirchoff, and M. P. Endress. "Altering Children's Distress Behavior During Orthopedic Cast Removal," *Nursing Research*, 24, no. 5 (November–December 1975), pp. 404–410.

Meleis, A. I., H. S. Wilson, and S. Chater. "Toward Scholarliness in Doctoral Dissertations: An Analytical Model," *Research in Nursing and Health*, 3, (1980), pp. 115–124.

19

Nonnurse Adult Students Return to School

Landra White, M.A.

Patricia Luna, Ed.S.

Adult students reentering the educational arena are in fact entering a different culture. This new culture demands different behavior from them than they may have previously practiced. The values and priorities may be different than those in familiar environments. All this results in anxiety, conflicting emotions, doubts about one's own ability and the value of the program, and multiple adjustments on the part of the student.

All adult students go through transitions. However, it has been our experience that adults in a large, multidisciplinary state university are different from nurses who return to nursing programs in several ways, and therefore the transition experiences may be somewhat different. Experienced nurses have successfully completed a postsecondary educational program, have had work experience in their field, and are pursuing further education in the same field in order to be successful or to advance within the field. Other adult students vary on all three of these factors. Many have no experience with college or postsecondary programs. Some attended one year "because my parents wanted me to; I wasn't really in school to learn anything and I didn't do well." Many people in this group are women who have been raising their children for the last several years.

Second, most adults in a university setting are not pursuing an education within a field for which they have already been trained. Many have no postsecondary training; others do not like their previous field. "I went into the military and became an electronic technician. I found I was completely disenchanted with the entire electronics field . . . . But while I was in, I discovered physical therapy and felt that would be a really good field for me." Some career changers have a specific goal; some are exploring. They do not experience the conflict with prior learning that nurses report. They do share with nurses some knowledge of "how the real world is" and, therefore, may experience conflict with the idealized world that education often presents.

Finally, not all adults are seeking an education to apply it to work. They may need a degree to advance, but do not necessarily expect the degree to be relevant to their work. They may be pursuing a degree "just to prove something to myself," or they may be exploring areas in which they have always been interested, but which they do not expect to use in earning a living. For example, one older woman had owned her own beauty shop for twenty years, but wanted to study art history. Thus nurses exhibit some differences from the larger population of adult college students. In general, adult college students enter higher education with backgrounds and motivations that lead to a wider variety of experiences, transitions, and adjustments than for a more homogeneous population such as nurses.

Nursing is highly structured. Most undergraduate fields do not have so structured a program as nursing. There are several specializations within business or engineering that are relatively structured, but still allow the student to experiment to find the area in which he or she fits best. The closest analogy to the clinical laboratories in nursing is the student teaching block in education. But education as a field lacks the quality of preciseness that characterizes the medical fields. The adult in a nursing program may have more of an impression of "there is only one right way and I don't know how to do it" than many other adults experience in their educational programs.

DO ADULT COLLEGE STUDENTS EXPERIENCE THE RETURNING-TO-SCHOOL SYNDROME?

In our work with adult college students, we have identified five distinct groups, sorted according to their prior educational experiences, current educational goals, and personal backgrounds. Utilizing the concepts of the returning-to-school syndrome (Shane, 1980), we will compare and contrast the experiences of these five groups as they return to school. The five groups are (1) the I've Never Been to College Group, (2) the I Need a Degree to Get Ahead Group, (3) the Changing Fields Group,

(4) the I Need a Credential in My Field Group, and (5) the I Want to Learn Group.

Our first observation is that few of the adult students we see experience a honeymoon. The size of the university, the unstructured aspects of the typical beginning curriculum, the students' lack of a clear goal, and the initial lack of contact with faculty in their chosen field makes the adult college student's return to school very anxiety provoking from the beginning.

Let's meet the five groups of adult college students.

Group One: I've Never Been to College

This is the largest single group of students we see. Most are women. Some women we include in this group actually have some prior college, but "it was a hundred years ago, I didn't know what I was doing, all I did was party and as a result I didn't do well at all." We cluster these two subgroups because their reactions are very similar.

The initial experience of this group to college is panic! "There was no honeymoon, unless your idea of a honeymoon is pretty awful." "It was very frightening; I was afraid of so many people, of not having any friends, of not being able to learn. A lot of women over thirty come into the university feeling that way." The anonymity of a large university is very intimidating. "I felt like I was not really here, like I could walk through people, like I was invisible, because I didn't feel like I was part of anything here at all. It was real scary."

The major characteristic of this group initially is vagueness. They may have little experience in decision making and often do not know what questions to ask. As a result, the questions they ask often appear irrelevant or trivial. For example, a liberal arts first-semester student may ask an advisor, "What am I supposed to take my first semester?," expecting an exact list that applies to all students. Since these questions often come in the busiest week of registration, the advisor may not be able to take time to explain all the factors that may affect those decisions. The student gets a brief answer and begins feeling "shuffled around from office to office." Such students quickly develop the impression that they are "stupid" and stop asking questions. The attitude of significant people in their lives may or may not be helpful and supportive. As they encounter additional requirements that they did not know about, they may decide "it's just not worth it."

Another example of vagueness is the lack of a clear goal. Many have finished raising their children "and now it's my turn to do something for myself." Some have gone through a divorce or widowhood and need to prepare for employment, "but I have no idea what I want to do."

The panic, aimlessness, and vagueness of goals seen in these students must be brought into some kind of perspective if they are to stay in school. Services in career exploration, decision making, and/or assertiveness techniques are frequently helpful.

The panic subsides as they find they can handle the work. Supportiveness of family and friends increases their confidence. But the single most critical factor seems to be finding other "older-than-average" students, not always an easy task for a part-time student at such a large university. Student associations are critical in developing a sense of belonging, gaining information, and learning the new skills needed for coping in this new culture.

If the aimlessness does not change, dropping out may be the best alternative. Rather than adding the frustrations of wasted time, these students often need to drop out in order to have time to define their priorities more clearly.

As they become more comfortable, the novice students enter a second stage. They seem to accept the structure and "go with the flow." "I'm feeling it out as I go; if I wind up with a degree, that's fantastic." After they realize they can choose from a wide variety of courses for their first two years, many view this favorably. "The first two years give you time to figure out a goal." Resentment of requirements is generally limited to specific requirements. "I'm angry about the Communications Skills Test requirement; the rest are just requirements and you do it."

Usually after they complete several semesters, the students enter a third stage; they begin to question the validity and relevance of their course work. They begin to wonder what application there could be for all this information. This questioning is common to most adult students. This group has no prior experience by which to measure their course work; they have neither academic nor practical standards. Similar to the young person, they have no point of reference; different from the young person, adults feel a time pressure to "get out and use all this." Unless these students begin to see practical application of their studies, they may drop out or postpone their degrees.

The fourth stage for this group is tailoring. They select a personal goal, and choose courses, professors, and projects related to their own goals or standards. Many of these students avail themselves of programs that have less structured requirements and that allow them to select their own courses. "I find that if I choose my courses correctly they are relevant to what I want to learn. I may take a class just for fun. But if I find I'm in a class that does not do anything for me, I drop it. That's how I deal with those situations."

Group Two: I Need a Degree to Get Ahead

These students have been working for some time and have decided that they are dead ended where they are. "I was in a job I was unhappy with. I felt I'd done all I could there. Also, I have been held up once or twice in my career by not having my piece of paper with 'bachelor of' on it." This group takes a very pragmatic approach; they are looking for courses that provide realistic information and practical skills. There is a definite feeling of time pressure; "returning students know time is money and the switch from 'your time is money' down to the college campus level of an easy loaf is a little bit hard to take." Most are also worried about their ability to "keep up with" the younger students academically.

The conflict stage comes very quickly for this group; in fact, they may enter college already in the conflict stage. Many anticipate or experience family conflicts before they enroll. Many also experience frustration at not being able to get specific, practical information about programs before they enter. Some enter college resentfully. They feel they are being required to spend a lot of time and money for "just a piece of paper." Some people in this group have already "been doing the boss's job." "Getting my passport is what this really is."

This group is likely to question requirements that do not seem related to their future job.

> I had to take eight hours of chemistry in order to be able to use ammonia to clean the [physical therapy] table. I asked the department chair who said it was a requirement from the national association. I wrote them and they sent me back a letter which [essentially] said "too bad, you have to take it anyway." But [at least] I tried to challenge the requirement.

> I think there are a lot of classes which aren't relevant, particularly the general liberal arts requirements which are set up like you are stupid, that you don't know what you want. If you come in knowing you want to be a psychologist, then there's no reason to take geology or astronomy. You should be able to direct your course load towards your major.

These students often quickly develop coping skills that we call *selective learning*. They set a standard for what they want to learn in a course and study to that level. "You cope with required courses by paying minimum attention to them, you pass with a C. The courses you're interested in, you'll spend much more time on and get better grades." One student gave this example:

> In an accounting course I was taking, the amount of time I would have had to spend to get an A would have been two to three hours a night. I wasn't willing to put in that amount of time. I was taking another class [in summer school] and working. I wanted to know how accounting worked, so that I

could supervise someone else doing bookkeeping; I didn't want to become an accountant myself. So I didn't do the homework, I just made a choice not to do homework and I just took a C in the course. I got what I wanted out of it and no more.

Their resentment usually diminishes if these students have set a goal and feel comfortable with that choice. For those in a relatively rigid program, the material will be more relevant and more meaningful as they get into the upper-level courses. They do not experience conflict with prior knowledge. "I've actually found that the things I'm learning in the classroom, in my area of concentration, complement my previous experiences. In fact what I have encountered is support for intuitions I've had, just based on gut feelings, rather than knowledge."

Focusing in on a personal goal positively resolves most of the conflict this group feels. They may still question some aspects of the curriculum, and they continue to question the usefulness and practical relevance of material. But they see the value of most of what they are learning. Thus, members of this group exhibit some aspects of the resolution stage of RTSS.

Group Three: Changing Fields—I Have a Degree But . . .

This group consists of people who have college degrees, but have decided their original field is no longer satisfactory. Some were teachers; others are those who have not been able to find jobs in their fields. The majority have been working and have become dissatisfied with their fields. This group may experience a honeymoon since they expect the new field will solve the problems and dissatisfactions they found in their previous field. Some expect the new field to cure their boredom, provide meaning in their lives, and produce other small miracles.

In leaving their previous field, these students have been undergoing a period of critical examination of themselves, their work, and the people they work with, both co-workers and supervisors. This examination has led them to leave their original field. However, as a result of this questioning process, they may exhibit a highly critical attitude. Some of these students are skeptical of ideas, challenge statements, and constantly search for flaws. If the new field does not stand up to the scrutiny, they become intensely disappointed and hostile. Their reaction is, "This is a farce. Why am I putting myself through this?" At the extreme, their anger is more vehement than the group who does not have degrees. They feel they have experienced *double* disappointments, and they are very angry.

Other students in this group do not experience such extreme disappointments. If they have had time to research their decision and to plan their transition to student status, they may be satisfied with the new knowledge.

For the angry students, there are several possible alternatives at this point. Some may drop out and go back to the old field, having realized that nothing is perfect. Others realize that they need more exploration and better decision making and take this opportunity to utilize career counseling services. These students may eventually change majors, continue in the new program, or drop out to pursue a field that does not require further education. The group that remains adjusts their standards toward being less idealistic and more practical.

Group Four: I Need a Credential in My Field

This group is a small percentage of the total adult student population. Their background and experiences are parallel to the nurse who returns to a nursing program. The returning-to-school syndrome generally describes their experiences quite well. They make contact with professors and staff who work in their specific field, and so are not overwhelmed by lack of direction. Since they have a specific goal, it is easier to make decisions and get information about appropriate courses. However, most of the students we see experience anxiety about their ability to succeed in college even prior to entering school.

In contrast to our other students, these students *do* experience conflict between their prior learning (whether an educational program or on-the-job training) and the new learning.

> I have to unlearn; I fight it. I've noticed a mental block, especially in bookkeeping which I've used on a practical basis. I find it harder to receive from the teacher or textbook. I find I'm saying "Oh, that's so ridiculous" because their theories are so wild. When I get into areas I don't know, I discover the teacher *is* teaching and the book *does* have something to say.

In some programs, these students make use of opportunities to avoid courses or teachers they consider irrelevant. Like the other groups of adult students, these students essentially "shop around" for coursework that is relevant to their individual goals. Professors who have practical experience and who can relate the theoretical knowledge to practical situations will find their classes full of "older-than-average" students. Universities will have to respond to the expectations of these students as the number of eighteen-year-old students declines.

Group Five: I've Got My Career—But I Still Want to Learn

This group explores areas for which there was no time before: lawyers study anthropology, managers explore sculpture. Their entire experience can be a honeymoon; they do not need practical information from their courses. They do not have to fulfill degree requirements. These people are enjoying the opportunity to fill in the gaps in their personal knowledge or experience.

Often these people exhibit a pattern of dropping in and dropping out. They attend class for one semester, then do not come back the next semester. The problems that these students encounter are primarily logistical; the lack of required prerequisites for a desired course seems to be a recurring problem. Since these students are not really in the educational culture, they experience little conflict or need for role adjustments.

General Observations

Our observation is that most adults returning to school experience frustrations, doubts, and a general loss of confidence. In their prior roles, they were usually in charge and knew the answers. In new roles, they must accept the answers provided by others. It apparently is natural to feel disoriented when the new role expected of an adult is different from more familiar roles.

Thoughts on Biculturalism

People who are actually bicultural (for example, members of minority ethnic groups who assume roles in the dominant culture), as in the more common usage of the term, have experiences similar to those described in RTSS. We believe, however, that in most cases it is not possible to incorporate all aspects of both cultures. For example, if you have been raised to be primarily a passive person, you may never be totally comfortable being a leader. If the values of the two cultures contradict each other, you cannot be both things at once. Shifting back and forth with the accompanying change of behavior can be stressful. The dilemma for the bicultural person often is to evaluate which aspects of *each* culture are most comfortable for that individual and to incorporate those aspects. This process requires an emotional distance from both cultures during which you feel very keenly that you do not quite fit into either culture.

SUMMARY

In summary, we frequently observe adult college students who question the validity of a new educational program and who retain doubts about the program for a long period of time. Adults have had many experiences that they have integrated, formulated informal theories that work for them, and developed ideas that have proved of worth in the real world. It is neither possible *nor desirable* to divest oneself of these "measuring sticks." On the other hand, being open to new knowledge is also important and necessary in this complex and changing world.

A questioning of your own ability is normal whether you are a nurse or any other sort of adult college student. When you push yourself beyond your previous level, you are taking a risk. Risks always entail the possibility of failure. Confidence comes after long experience in a particular situation or role. In terms of education, confidence in your ability to perform what you have been taught may come only after you have returned to the job and practiced your knowledge for some time.

Your family and friends play a crucial role in the initial process of working through feelings of doubt and fear. If they can be supportive and take some of the day-to-day load off your shoulders, you will have less stress. But it may be that you find yourself in a situation of being a single parent to three young children. This situation may present such an enormous strain on you that you cannot continue in your present educational program. This does not mean that you are a failure or will never be able to complete your degree. It simply means that you are human, that you have other commitments, and that this was not the right time for this program in your life.

We believe that adult students who experience less than full acceptance of a program are valuable students. Full acceptance of an educational program is a goal that sounds very attractive. "If only I was sure this was right for me," is a frequently heard lament. However, for an adult, full acceptance would mean that there would be no room to contribute an individual perspective, a different viewpoint, or new information that might not fit the "model." Full acceptance by all students would mean that the educational program would not grow and develop. These results would not be productive for either the students or the program.

Questioning and doubts are apparently necessary by-products of any personal growth. As you make your own transitions, it may help to know that other nonnurse students experience similar transitions.

REFERENCES

For additional references on adult learners, see the References at the end of Chapter 13.

Shane, Donea L. "The Returning to School Syndrome," in *Teaching Tomorrow's Nurse: A Nurse Educator Reader*, ed. S. K. Mirin. Wakefield, Mass.: Nursing Resources, Inc., 1980.

Index